The

Molecular

Foundations

of

Psychiatry

The

Molecular

Foundations

of

Psychiatry

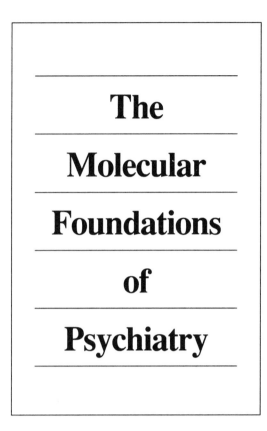

Steven E. Hyman, M.D.
Director, Division on Addictions
Harvard Medical School
Assistant Professor of Psychiatry and Neuroscience
Massachusetts General Hospital and Harvard Medical School
Boston, Massachusetts

Eric J. Nestler, M.D., Ph.D.
Director, Division of Molecular Psychiatry
Elizabeth Mears and House Jameson Associate Professor
of Psychiatry and Pharmacology
Connecticut Mental Health Center and Yale University School of Medicine
New Haven, Connecticut

American Psychiatric Press, Inc.

Washington, DC
London, England

Note: The authors have worked to ensure that all information in this book concerning drug dosages, schedules, and routes of administration is accurate as of the time of publication and consistent with standards set by the U.S. Food and Drug Administration and the general medical community. As medical research and practice advance, however, therapeutic standards may change. For this reason and because human and mechanical errors sometimes occur, we recommend that readers follow the advice of a physician who is directly involved in their care or the care of a member of their family.

Books published by the American Psychiatric Press, Inc., represent the views and opinions of the individual authors and do not necessarily represent the policies and opinions of the Press or the American Psychiatric Association.

Copyright © 1993 American Psychiatric Press, Inc.
ALL RIGHTS RESERVED
Manufactured in the United States of America on acid-free paper
96 95 94 93   4 3 2
First Edition

American Psychiatric Press, Inc.
1400 K Street, N.W., Washington, DC   20005

Library of Congress Cataloging-in-Publication Data
Hyman, Steven E.
    The Molecular foundations of psychiatry / Steven E. Hyman, Eric J.
Nestler. — 1st ed.
        p. cm.
    Includes bibliographical references and index.
    ISBN 0-88048-353-9
    1. Neuropsychiatry. 2. Neuropsychopharmacology. 3. Mental
illness—Molecular aspects. 4. Mental illness—Genetic aspects.
I. Title.
    [DNLM: 1. Mental Disorders—etiology. 2. Mental Disorders—
genetics. 3. Molecular Biology. 4. Neurobiology.
5. Neuropharmacology. 6. Neuropsychology.   WM 100 H996m]
RC341.H96   1993
616.8—dc20
DNLM/DLC
for Library of Congress   92-7017
                                                                      CIP

British Library Cataloguing in Publication Data
A CIP record is available from the British Library.

Contents

3 | OVERVIEW OF NEUROPSYCHOPHARMACOLOGY   55

4 | MECHANISMS OF NEURAL PLASTICITY   95

5 | DRUG-INDUCED NEURAL PLASTICITY: HOW PSYCHOTROPIC DRUGS WORK   123

6 | OVERVIEW OF PSYCHIATRIC GENETICS   173

7 | TOWARD A NEW PSYCHIATRIC NEUROSCIENCE   193

Preface

Called a "Disease of the Mind," it afflicts more than one-third of patients in mental institutions. A severely debilitating and chronic illness affecting diverse aspects of higher brain function, it causes impaired cognition, distorted perceptions, and hallucinations. Highly resistant to standard treatments, it can present abruptly in healthy individuals or develop insidiously over a long period. Those afflicted with the disease are stigmatized because society views the illness as caused by breakdowns in morality and in the family structure.[*]

This account of neurosyphilis given close to 100 years ago could be used to describe schizophrenia today. We are perplexed by the etiology of schizophrenia and frustrated by our limited ability to treat its manifestations or alter its long-term course. The above description also illustrates how our ignorance can lead to gross misconceptions and sometimes almost magical accounts of disease pathogenesis.

A great debate continues within the field of psychiatry as to its central philosophy and orientation. There are struggles between "biological" and "psychological" explanations and treatments for illnesses. There is also a growing perception that we have reached roadblocks in our ability to treat severely disabled patients. With few exceptions, most of the available treatments for mental disorders were discovered serendipitously, have been around for decades, and, although effective for many patients, have serious side effects. In addition, a core of patients remain who are relatively unresponsive. These individuals with treatment-resistant disorders and their families face long-term disability and suffering, and society faces ever-escalating costs. At the same time, public and private funds available for treatment appear to be diminishing. Psychiatry is at a crossroads.

Virtually all illnesses have biological, psychological, and social dimensions, including common medical illnesses such as diabetes, tuberculosis, cancer, and heart disease. Ultimately, however, it is the biological understanding of a disease, an understanding of its pathophysiology, that leads to definitive treat-

---

[*]Paraphrased from Brandt AM: "The Syphilis Epidemic and Its Relation to AIDS." *Science* 239:375–380, 1988; and Korenman SG: "The Problems of Substance Abuse," in *UCLA/NIDA Symposium on Substance Abuse*. Edited by Korenman SG, Barchas JD. New York, Oxford University Press (in press).

ment and prevention. Tuberculosis is an example of a disorder in which an understanding of the biology led to a shift from less effective social interventions (i.e., recuperation in a sanitarium) to potent pharmacological interventions (i.e., antibiotics).

However, an understanding of the biological basis of a disease does not necessarily diminish the role of psychological and social treatments. An understanding of the pathophysiology may even lead to effective behavioral interventions for some disorders. For example, phenylketonuria, a major cause of mental retardation decades ago, was found to be the result of a genetic mutation in a single enzyme. This biological information led to an essentially behavioral, but effective, approach to the disorder: all clinical symptoms of the illness can be prevented by avoidance of dietary phenylalanine. In the prevention and treatment of heart disease, behavioral interventions—cessation of smoking and increased exercise—are generally combined with pharmacological interventions.

Although treatments for many medical disorders have been developed empirically without detailed pathophysiological knowledge, progress in such situations is generally haphazard and limited. In contrast, a detailed knowledge of pathophysiology allows the development of multiple, often complementary, approaches to a disorder, yielding a high likelihood that everyone can be treated. A good example is the treatment of peptic ulcer, which can be approached rationally with H_2 receptor antagonists, H^+ ion pump inhibitors, antibiotics, prostaglandins, agents that coat the gastric mucosa, or antacids, or with some combination of these agents. The upshot is that effective treatment with minimal side effects can be provided for almost everyone, and ulcer surgery (an additional treatment of last resort) has become extremely rare.

There is nothing unique about mental disorders in this regard. They also have biological, psychological, and social dimensions. Much clinical psychiatry now focuses appropriately on psychosocial rehabilitative measures, as direct interventions targeted to the underlying abnormalities of the disorders are usually unavailable. We need to improve these rehabilitative measures to help patients compensate better for their impairments and maximize their ability to function. At the same time, however, we must redouble our efforts to learn more about the diseases of the brain that lead to these perplexing mental disorders. Through such neurobiological research, more definitive and effective treatments will be devised.

As the pathophysiology of these disturbances is identified over the next several decades, we are confident that the practice of psychiatry will change radically in the way it approaches psychotic, affective, anxiety, substance abuse, and other disorders. This will surely be a difficult task, given the likely involvement of complex etiological factors, and will require considerable time and resources, but the difficulty of the task cannot detract from the importance of the goal—only through a greater understanding of the basic molecular and neurobiological mechanisms involved in major psychiatric disorders will it be possible to greatly advance the field of psychiatry. Years from now, relatively clear-cut explanations for these disorders will be striking compared with our 1990s confusion, just as identification of the *Treponema* spirochete revolutionized our view of neurosyphilis.

The objective of this book, then, is to review recent findings in basic molecular biology and the basic neurosciences that establish the foundations of a molecular approach to psychiatry. Molecular studies in psychiatry are aimed at identifying the precise molecular substrates (i.e., individual genes and proteins) through which diverse types of genetic and environmental factors combine to produce specific disease states. However, before specific hypotheses concerning the molecular basis of gene-environment interactions can be considered (in Chapter 7), considerable attention must be given first to basic molecular biology and basic neuropharmacology, which provide the foundations for these hypotheses. Thus, the primary focus of the earlier chapters of the text is neural transmission, the regulation of gene expression in the brain, and the intracellular messenger pathways in the brain that provide the causal bridges between environmental stimuli and the control of neural gene expression. This emphasis on gene expression and mechanisms underlying persistent changes in brain function makes sense given the importance of long-term adaptive phenomena in both the onset and recovery from most forms of mental illness.

The new information derived from molecular investigations in psychiatry will revolutionize the field by leading to the development of improved diagnostic and prognostic tests, to new and more effective treatments, and ultimately to the development of preventive measures.

Introduction

Psychiatric research is uniquely difficult. The human brain, the organ on which psychiatric research must focus, is the most complex structure in all of biology. Despite advances in neuroimaging technologies, the living human brain remains largely inaccessible for study. Moreover, because of the uniqueness of the human brain, human behavior, and, presumably, human consciousness, satisfactory animal models of psychiatric disorders are lacking. Even psychiatric research that does not directly involve the brain, such as psychiatric genetics, has been confounded because the boundaries separating psychiatric disorders from each other and, in some cases, separating disorder from normality are often unclear. Despite these difficulties, the tools of modern neuroscience and of molecular genetics promise unparalleled advances in the coming decades in our understanding of the pathophysiology of psychiatric disorders and of the mechanisms of action of psychotropic drugs and even, perhaps, of psychotherapies.

To make progress, however, these tools must be used well. Molecular genetic linkage analyses of psychiatric disorders can only be successful if phenotypic classification of patients is improved and better human genetic strategies are employed. Better strategies are also needed in the basic neuroscience of psychiatry. For the last three decades, mainstream biological research in psychiatry has been focused excessively, in part by necessity, on simplistic pharmacological approaches to the brain. Much of this research approached the nervous system as if it were an endocrine organ in which too much or too little of a given neurotransmitter were responsible for a disease state. The most common measures of brain function used in this approach are determination of steady-state or pharmacologically stimulated levels of neurotransmitters and hormones, measurement of neurotransmitter metabolites as markers of neurotransmitter turnover, and measurement of neurotransmitter receptor sensitivity either from receptor binding studies in brain homogenates or inferred from physiological responses to drugs administered to human subjects.

However, the brain cannot be understood in the context of an endocrinological-pharmacological model that ignores the complex connectivity of the brain and its diverse cellular signaling mechanisms. The inadequacy of such an approach can be illustrated by attempts over the years to study the "serotonergic" or "dopaminergic" systems in the brain in terms of serotonin or dopamine turnover as measured by neurotransmitter levels or metabolites in some body fluid.

Both serotonin and dopamine are utilized by multiple neural projection systems with markedly different functions. Moreover, changes induced in a single neural projection system, for example, in response to a particular pharmacological agent, probably lead to numerous, sometimes reciprocal, changes elsewhere that may not be predictable a priori. This complexity means that, for much of the psychopharmacological data currently available, it is difficult to argue that putative neurotransmitter and receptor abnormalities provide insight into the pathophysiology of psychiatric disorders, rather than being consequences that may be quite far removed from the disease etiology in the chain of connections.

Problems with the endocrinological-pharmacological approach to the brain extend beyond their inability to account for neural projection systems. To return to the examples of serotonin and dopamine, there are numerous types of receptors for each of these two neurotransmitters. The different receptors for a given neurotransmitter can have very different consequences for signaling within the receiving neuron. For example, the effect of serotonin binding on one target neuron may be the opposite of its effect on another. From this point of view, phrases that are often used in the psychopharmacological literature, such as "the serotonin system" or "serotonergic tone," are too imprecise to offer accurate information about the pathophysiology of psychiatric disorders or the mechanism of action of psychotropic drugs.

To improve our understanding of disease pathophysiology and drug action, the endocrinological-pharmacological paradigm, which was by and large the most feasible approach until recently, should be supplanted by newly developed paradigms made possible by advances in modern neuroscience and molecular biology. First, greater attention must be paid to the function of particular neural projections and to their interactions with each other. This is sometimes referred to as "systems neurobiology" or the "top-down approach" to the brain. This approach attempts to identify particular neural systems that underlie various physiological outputs, including behavior. The major tools of this approach are those of the neuroanatomist and electrophysiologist. Combined with such a systems approach, pharmacological analyses gain a new precision. Obviously, pending major advances in neuroimaging technologies, this approach is largely limited to animal studies.

Second, greater attention must be given to what can be called cellular and molecular neurobiology or the "bottom-up approach." This approach, which has produced extraordinary advances in neurobiology during the past decade, is the focus of this book. The tools of cellular and molecular neurobiology are largely those of the biochemist and molecular biologist, although electrophysiological tools, such as those permitting the measurement of ion fluxes, are also required.

The endocrinological-pharmacological approach to psychiatric research fo-

cused largely on synaptic function and ignored the events that occurred within
neurons. In essence, it stopped at the receptor and treated the neuron as a black
box. However, the observations that the therapeutic effects of most of the important classes of psychotropic drugs (lithium and antidepressant, antipsychotic,
and atypical anxiolytic agents) generally take weeks to develop and that states
of addiction generally require multiple exposures to a drug suggest strongly that
it is not the initial synaptic targets of these drugs that are critically important,
but rather the slow-onset adaptive changes that occur within neurons in response
to those initial interactions. Similar types of long-term changes in neural function must underlie memory and, in all likelihood, the pervasive state changes
observed in such disease states as mood and psychotic disorders. Such long-term
changes in neural function can only be understood if psychiatry supplements its
traditional interest in synaptic pharmacology with in-depth research at the cellular and molecular level. The primary goal of this book is to provide an introduction to modern cellular neuroscience and molecular biology as they are
relevant to psychiatry.

In Chapter 1, we offer an introduction to proteins and nucleic acids, the key
molecular components of cells, including basic reviews of their synthesis and
regulation. We review in Chapter 2 the biology of the synapse, with an emphasis
on neurotransmitters, receptors, and postreceptor signal transduction pathways
found within the brain. In Chapter 3, we present an overview of neuropharmacology that focuses on the acute actions that psychotropic drugs exert on brain
function via their interactions with neurotransmitters, receptors, and the like. In
Chapter 4, we present the types of mechanisms that are now known to underlie
long-term changes in the nervous system. Chapter 5 represents a progress report
of ongoing research aimed at explaining how psychotropic drugs produce their
clinically important effects on the brain, that is, their delayed-onset, long-term
effects. The view presented is that such long-term effects represent, in essence,
drug-induced neural plasticity. As will be seen in Chapters 4 and 5, two major
types of mechanisms are likely to be of paramount importance to psychiatric
neuroscience: protein phosphorylation and the regulation of neuronal gene expression. In Chapter 6, we provide an overview of psychiatric genetics with
particular attention to molecular approaches.

Because many of the molecular processes described in the earlier chapters of
the book function to transduce signals from the environment into changes in
neuronal function, the study of molecular neurobiology suggests mechanisms by
which experience and other environmental inputs interact with neurons and even
the genome. In Chapter 7, we explore such molecular mechanisms, some of
which remain hypothetical, and discuss experimental strategies by which these
mechanisms can be investigated in the future.

Chapter 7 thereby embodies a second major aim of our book, to reflect on the implications of modern molecular neuroscience for dichotomies between so-called biological and so-called psychological approaches to psychiatry. These dichotomies, so prominent in recent psychiatric thinking, are evident in discussions of whether a particular psychological trait or mental disorder reflects the influence of genes (nature) or environment (nurture) and whether it involves the brain (and is therefore "biological") or the mind (and is therefore "psychological"). We hope to make it clear that brain function is neither the deterministic product of genes unfolding in a vacuum, nor of environmental influences imprinted on a tabula rasa, but, rather, the result of complex gene-environment interactions about which some details are beginning to emerge. Indeed, we will show that interactions between the environment and the genome do not end with birth, but continue throughout life. Moreover, we hope by the end of the book to make it clear that the strong Cartesian position that has typified so much psychiatric discussion (i.e., a denial of substantial and important causal interactions between the brain and genetics on the one hand and the environment and psychological experience on the other) makes no sense. Psychological and neurobiological explanations represent different approaches to the same substrate—the brain. Experiences and, of course, psychotherapy itself can only be processed and have an effect on an individual insofar as they influence neurons. Although the nature of consciousness may remain a philosophical problem, how experience influences the brain is an empirical question, which can be approached in a meaningful way using the tools provided by modern neurobiology.

We have strived throughout the book to provide a clear overview of the material, without sacrificing so much detail as to render the discussion empty. In each chapter, the material presented starts at a beginning level that requires little prior knowledge of the field and develops gradually to a considerably sophisticated level. This more detailed material, indicated throughout by vertical rules in the left margin of text, can be skipped by individuals interested in a more general overview of the field, without loss of the overall message of the book. With this organization, the book can be used both as an introduction for practicing clinical psychiatrists to a fundamentally new body of knowledge in psychiatry and as a text of the basic neuroscience of psychiatry for psychiatric residents, medical and graduate students, senior undergraduates, and academic psychiatrists.

The book need not be read cover to cover. The individual chapters are somewhat self-sufficient so that individuals interested in a particular area can go directly to the relevant chapter. The book can thereby also serve as a reference guide to the basic neuroscience of psychiatry. In this regard, we should mention that individuals particularly interested in an overview of "molecular psychiatry" may wish to read the final chapter (Chapter 7) first and then refer to earlier chapters to obtain the necessary background information, which would clearly depend a great deal on their prior knowledge of basic molecular neurobiology. Finally, no attempt is made in the book to provide detailed references for the numerous scientific findings presented. Instead, a small number of review articles and selected primary references are given at the end of each chapter. Readers should realize that research in the areas described is extremely active; this text should be only the starting point for their pursuit of this field.

We would like to thank the following individuals for their inspiration and helpful discussions during recent years: Drs. Ronald S. Duman, Gerald Fischbach, Edwin Furshpan, David Potter, George R. Heninger, Larry H. Price, and Bruce M. Cohen. We would like to thank those who read and critiqued drafts of the chapters, especially Dr. Deborah Blacker, and would also like to acknowledge our residents and students, whose curiosity stimulated the writing of this text.

Chapter 1

Introduction to

Molecular Biology

This chapter introduces the major molecular components of cells. In much of the remainder of the book, we explain important aspects of brain function and the action of psychotropic drugs on the basis of the molecular building blocks described here. From the point of view of understanding the molecular biology of psychiatry, it is less important to learn all of the details presented here than to come away with an overview of the functions of the basic macromolecules of cells and a conception of how their synthesis is regulated.

NUCLEIC ACIDS AND PROTEINS

The most important building blocks of cells are two classes of macromolecules: the nucleic acids (deoxyribonucleic acid—DNA—and ribonucleic acid—RNA) and proteins. This chapter offers a simple overview of what these two types of macromolecules are, how they are synthesized, and how they appear to be involved in virtually every aspect of cellular function.

Nucleic Acids

The structure of DNA, which was determined by Watson and Crick in 1953, is a helix composed of two strands. Each of the strands is a linear molecule composed of small building blocks called nucleotides. The genetic information that is contained by DNA is coded by the linear sequence of these nucleotides. A *nucleotide* consists of a nitrogen-containing ring group (a purine or pyrimidine) joined to a sugar group (deoxyribose or ribose), with a phosphate group at-

---

Text defined by vertical rules in the left margin involves advanced concepts and can be skipped by readers interested in a more general overview of the field, without loss of the overall message of the book.

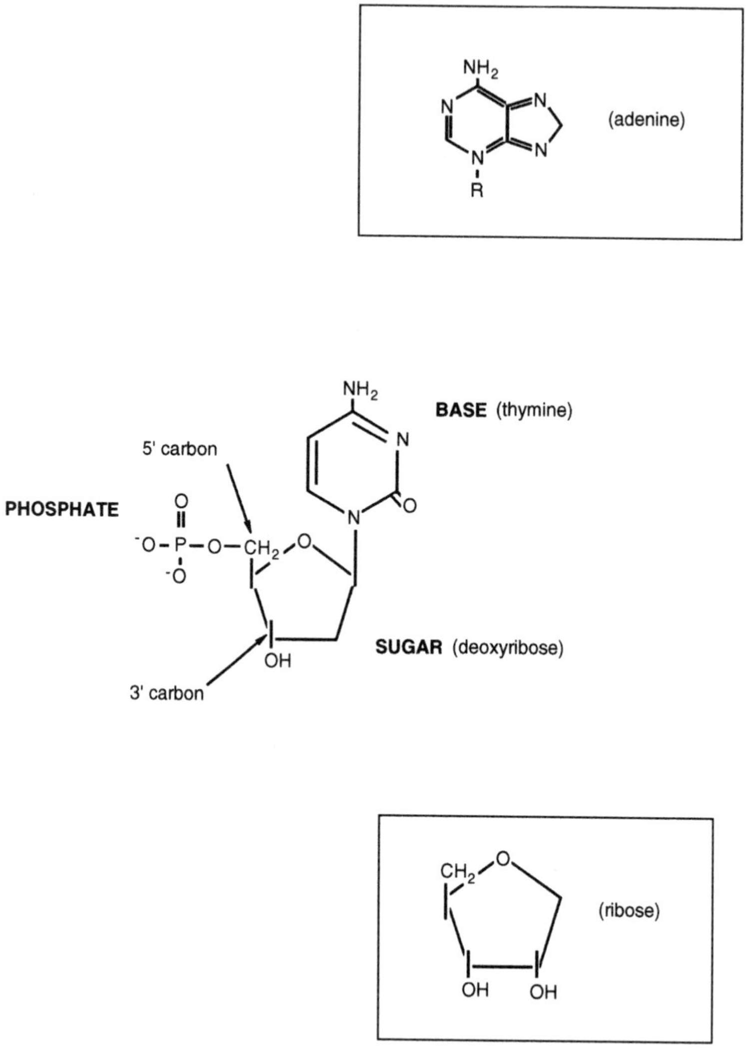

FIGURE 1–1.   **Chemical structure of a nucleotide.** The nucleotide deoxythymidine-5'-monophosphate is illustrated. It is composed of the pyrimidine base thymine, the sugar deoxyribose, and a phosphate group. Illustrated in the *upper box* for comparison is the purine base adenine. Illustrated in the *lower box* is the sugar ribose, which is a component of RNA. Ribose differs from deoxyribose by having a hydroxyl group on its 2' carbon. The 5' and 3' carbons of deoxyribose that form bonds with phosphate groups in nucleic acids are illustrated. (Insets are not to scale.)

tached to the sugar (Figure 1–1). The purine or pyrimidine itself is called a *base;* a base joined to a sugar group is called a *nucleoside;* and a phosphorylated nucleoside is called a *nucleotide.* DNA and RNA are each synthesized out of four types of nucleotide bases. The four nucleotides that make up DNA are the deoxyribose forms of the purines—adenine (A) and guanine (G)—and the pyrimidines—cytosine (C) and thymine (T). The four nucleotides that make up RNA are the ribose forms of adenine, guanine, and cytosine and the pyrimidine uracil (U) (which takes the place of thymine in RNA).

Individual nucleotides are joined into strands of DNA or RNA via the phosphate groups: the phosphate groups form ester bonds with the 5′ carbon on the sugar group of one nucleotide and the 3′ carbon on a sugar group of a second nucleotide and so on (Figure 1–2). This phosphodiester linkage of the 5′ carbon of one sugar to the 3′ carbon of the next gives individual strands of DNA and RNA an intrinsic directionality that, as will be seen, is biologically significant. The end of a DNA strand with a free (unbound) 5′ carbon on the sugar group of its terminal base is termed the *5′ end* of the strand and the other end with a free 3′ carbon is termed the *3′ end;* by convention DNA sequences are written from 5′ to 3′.

The two strands of the double helix are said to be antiparallel to each other in that the 5′ end of one strand is opposite the 3′ end of the other. The alternating deoxyribose sugar and phosphate groups that connect the bases of each strand

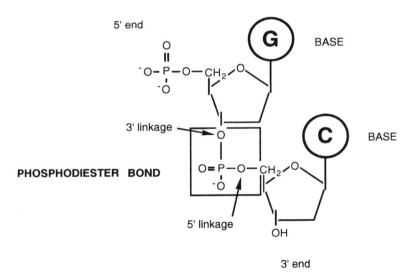

FIGURE 1–2. Chemical structure of a dinucleotide illustrating a phosphodiester bond, which forms the backbone of the DNA helix (see text).

form what is called a "sugar-phosphate backbone" on the outside of the double helix. All of the bases of the DNA molecule are found on the inside of the double helix (Figure 1–3). The bases from each strand are apposed very closely to each other. The double helix fits together only if a large purine base (A or G) is across from a smaller pyrimidine base (T or C). As shown in Figure 1–1, a purine contains two rings, a pyrimidine only one. In fact, the nucleotide base A is always across from (or paired with) T, and G is paired with C. This situation is described by stating that A is complementary to T, and G is complementary to C (Figure 1–4).

Such "base pairing" is due to the fact that only pairs of complementary nucleotides form a maximum number of stabilizing hydrogen bonds. Any other arrangement of bases destabilizes the structure of the DNA. As will be seen later in this chapter, the principle of complementary base pairing forms the basis of DNA replication and RNA transcription. Complementary base pairing also enables molecular biologists to detect the presence of a particular DNA or RNA sequence: under the right conditions, a radioactively labeled fragment of DNA or RNA (called a probe) will form a double helix only with its complement; this permits the detection of complementary strands, even within complex mixtures of DNAs and RNAs. This process of annealing of radiolabeled probes to complementary strands is called *hybridization*.

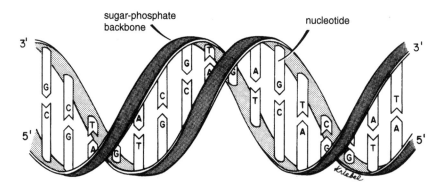

FIGURE 1–3. The double helix of DNA. Two complementary strands of DNA hybridize with one another to form a double helix. The two strands of a double helix are oriented in opposite directions (antiparallel): the 3′ end of one is across from the 5′ end of the other. The sugar-phosphate backbones of the two strands are found on the outside of the double helix; the bases are found on the inside. Formation of a DNA double helix is stabilized when hydrogen bonds form between complementary bases of the two strands. Two hydrogen bonds form when A is across from T; three hydrogen bonds form when G is across from C. Other appositions of bases are destabilizing and do not occur.

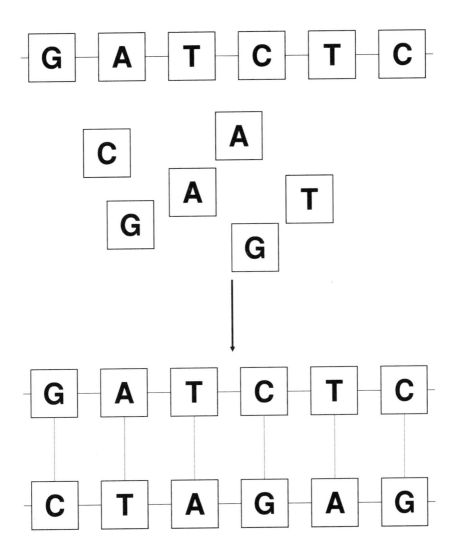

FIGURE 1–4. Schematic illustration of complementary base pairing. A strand of DNA can serve as a template for a second strand of nucleic acid (DNA or RNA). A polymerase enzyme assembles individual nucleotides into a new strand using the first strand as a template. The sequence of the new strand is therefore determined by the template. In addition, based on the principle of complementary base pairing, single nucleic acid strands that are complementary to each other will hybridize with each other under experimental conditions. The better the match (i.e., complementarity) between the two strands, the stronger the hybridization will be. Many molecular biological procedures take advantage of such hybridization reactions.

The major function of DNA is to carry the genetic blueprint of the cell. This is true for all living organisms, including prokaryotes (i.e., bacteria and blue-green algae) and eukaryotes (i.e., all animals, protozoa, fungi, and plants). One major difference between eukaryotic and prokaryotic cells is that all the hereditary material (DNA) of eukaryotic cells is contained in a distinct subcellular organelle, the nucleus. Throughout the evolutionary tree, cells carry DNA as extremely extended molecules, known as chromosomes, which contain thousands of genes. In addition to containing genes, chromosomes of eukaryotic organisms also contain much additional DNA, of unknown function, interspersed among the genes.

Within nuclei, chromosomes are packaged with a set of proteins called *histones* into a relatively amorphous material called *chromatin*. It is thought that DNA in chromatin is relatively loosely packed so as to allow genes to function. Individual chromosomes become visible by microscopy only when they condense as a cell begins to divide. Such condensation is probably necessary for efficient and complete replication of the chromosomes and segregation of chromosomes into the daughter cells.

As will be seen, the polynucleotide structure of DNA is well suited for the storage of information and for self-replication, but its chemical simplicity and its relatively rigid helical structure limit the number of functions that DNA can perform in the cell. From an evolutionary point of view this may be why the information contained within DNA is expressed through two other molecules—RNAs and proteins.

Like DNA, RNA is chemically quite simple (composed of four nucleotides), but because it is a nonrigid single strand and free to fold into a variety of conformations, it is somewhat more functionally versatile than DNA. Messenger RNA (mRNA) functions as an intermediary between the sequence of DNA and the sequence of proteins. As in the case of DNA, mRNA carries information encoded in its linear sequence of nucleotides. Other RNA molecules serve structural purposes in cells, however. Ribosomes, the organelles on which proteins are synthesized, are constructed out of complexes of ribosomal RNA (rRNA) and proteins. Another structural RNA, transfer RNA (tRNA), serves to deliver specific amino acids to ribosomes for incorporation into proteins during the process of protein synthesis.

As described above, RNA has two minor chemical differences from DNA, in addition to being single stranded: the sugar phosphate backbone of RNA contains the sugar ribose instead of deoxyribose, and the base thymine (T) is replaced by uracil (U). U is structurally quite similar to T and is also complementary to A.

Proteins

Proteins, like nucleic acids, are linear polymers; they are single unbranched chains of amino acid building blocks. An *amino acid* is a small molecule that contains an amino group (NH_2) and a carboxylic acid or carboxy group (COOH) plus a variable side chain in between (Figures 1–5 and 1–6). Individual amino acids are linked by peptide bonds, whereby the amino group of one amino acid is joined to the carboxy group of another amino acid. This gives proteins an intrinsic orientation, with one end of the protein containing a free amino terminus and the other containing a free carboxy terminus. Because proteins are joined by peptide bonds, they are often described as *peptides* or *polypeptides,* although these terms are usually reserved for relatively small proteins, that is, short amino acid chains.

Proteins are constructed from 20 kinds of amino acids. By incorporating so many different amino acids, each with their chemically diverse side chains (diverse in size, shape, hydrophobicity, and charge), proteins have much greater functional versatility than either DNA or RNA. The specific properties of proteins depend not only on the linear sequence of their amino acid building blocks (primary structure), but also on their folded three-dimensional characteristics (secondary and tertiary structure). In addition, proteins may fold into structures involving more than one amino acid chain (quaternary structure). In such cases the individual chains are called *subunits.*

Cells contain hundreds of thousands of distinct proteins, each with unique structural and functional properties. Indeed, individual proteins function in markedly different ways and subserve virtually every aspect of cell function. There are structural proteins that serve as cytoskeletal components of cells and thereby determine the highly specialized shapes of cells and the transport of subcellular components within them. Enzymes are proteins that catalyze and

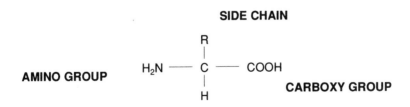

SIDE CHAIN

AMINO GROUP

$$H_2N \longrightarrow \underset{\underset{H}{|}}{\overset{\overset{R}{|}}{C}} \longrightarrow COOH$$

CARBOXY GROUP

FIGURE 1–5. Amino acid chemical structure. The amino acid building blocks of proteins are chemically varied, but all contain an amino group and a carboxylic acid (or carboxy) group. Each of the 20 amino acids found in proteins has a distinct side chain, shown as *R* in the figure.

regulate virtually all of the chemical reactions that occur within cells and thereby determine the other chemical constituents of cells. Ion channels and transmembrane transporters are proteins that regulate the flow of ions and small

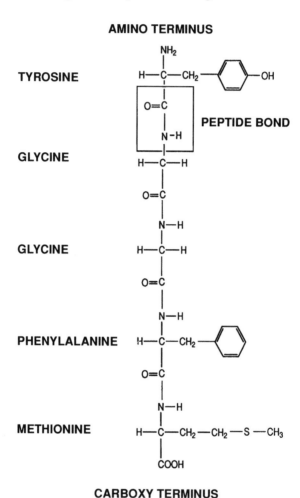

FIGURE 1–6. Chemical structure of a small polypeptide: Met-enkephalin. A protein is a linear polymer of amino acids joined by a series of peptide bonds formed between the carboxy group of one amino acid and the amino group of the next *(box)*. The peptide (small protein) shown in the figure (Tyr-Gly-Gly-Phe-Met) is the opioid neurotransmitter Met-enkephalin. Just as nucleic acids can be described directionally (see Figure 1–2), proteins have an intrinsic direction: one end contains a free amino group and is termed the *amino terminus*, whereas the other end contains a free carboxy group and is termed the *carboxy terminus*.

molecules across cell membranes. As will be discussed in Chapter 2, receptors and G proteins (so named because of their ability to bind guanine nucleotides) are proteins that control the flow of information from the outside to the inside of cells. Even certain intercellular messengers are small proteins (peptides), including growth factors, cytokines, neuropeptides, and a subset of hormones.

DNA REPLICATION

A critical property of a linear polymer such as DNA (or RNA) is that it can serve as a template for the synthesis of other macromolecules (Figure 1–4). In the case of nucleic acids, the principle of complementary base pairing provides the mechanism by which information can be transferred across generations. Because each strand of the DNA double helix contains a nucleotide sequence that is the exact complement of the sequence of its partner, both strands contain the same information. Each strand can therefore serve as a template for the synthesis of a complementary strand also containing the same information.

The actual enzymatic steps involved in the replication of DNA are quite complex, but the overall principles can be stated quite simply. Replication begins with separation of the two complementary DNA strands in a local region. Each strand then serves as a template for a new DNA molecule by the sequential polymerization of nucleotides. This reaction is catalyzed in the 5' to 3' direction by an enzyme called DNA polymerase; the enzyme adds a new nucleotide base to the 3' end of the growing DNA chain. Selection of the correct base to be added at each step depends on its being complementary to the next base in the parental template strand. Eventually the replication process generates two complete DNA double helices, each identical in sequence to the original. DNA replication is said to be *semiconservative* because each daughter DNA molecule contains one of the original parental strands plus one newly synthesized strand.

The energy for adding each successive new phosphodiester bond is derived from the incoming nucleotides themselves. Nucleotides enter the reaction as deoxyribonucleoside triphosphates. Only one phosphate is required for the phosphodiester bond; the remaining pyrophosphate can be hydrolyzed with the release of energy.

INFORMATION FLOWS FROM DNA TO RNA TO PROTEIN

Geneticists initially had difficulty accepting DNA as the physical basis of heredity, because it is chemically so simple (i.e., an unbranched polymer of only four subunits). However, in addition to explaining DNA replication, the structure of DNA also explains how it can store information. DNA carries information by means of the linear sequence of its nucleotides. Based on experiments with mutated DNA (DNA in which the nucleotide sequence is altered), it was determined that DNA and protein are colinear—that is, the nucleotides in a particular sequence of DNA are arranged in an order corresponding to the order of the amino acids in the protein they specify. It was determined empirically that each linear sequence of three nucleotides specifies a single amino acid. The particular amino acid specified by any grouping of three nucleotides is called the *genetic code.*

As a first approximation, a gene is a region of DNA that codes for the synthesis of a single protein, although, as will be discussed later in this chapter, differential processing of RNA can introduce some variety into the protein products of a single gene. In addition to a region that codes for proteins, genes also contain DNA sequences that determine in what tissues and under what circumstances the gene will be active.

Proteins are not synthesized directly from DNA that encodes them, however, but rather in two sequential processes—*transcription* of DNA into mRNA, which occurs in the nucleus, and *translation* of the mRNA into protein, which occurs in the cytoplasm.

Conceptually, transcription is similar to DNA replication in that one of the two strands of DNA serves as a template to produce an exact complement in terms of nucleotide sequence. However, instead of producing a second strand of nucleic acid that remains annealed to the template strand (as in DNA replication), transcription produces an RNA strand that is released from the template. This allows the DNA of the gene to reform the double helix and the RNA, which remains single stranded, to be further processed and then to exit the nucleus for translation. Because it is an exact complement of the gene, the mRNA produced by transcription retains all of the information of the DNA sequence from which it was synthesized. Synthesis of mRNA by DNA transcription, like DNA replication, always proceeds in the 5' to 3' direction.

Transcription of DNA Into RNA

The process of transcription can be divided into three steps: initiation, elongation of the transcript, and termination. Although many levels of regulation are important, transcription initiation appears to be the major control point gating the flow of information from the genome. It will therefore be described in detail.

In eukaryotes, transcription of genes that encode proteins (as opposed to structural RNAs such as rRNA or tRNA) is carried out by the enzyme RNA polymerase II and associated regulatory proteins. These regulatory proteins form complexes with the polymerase (termed a *polymerase II complex*) and play critical roles in regulating the two aspects of transcription initiation that are required for accurate transcription: First, RNA polymerase II must be positioned at the correct transcriptional start sites of genes, and second, the rate of transcription initiations must be controlled to produce the appropriate amount of a particular mRNA for the cell's needs.

The proteins that are involved in regulating transcription are called *transcription factors,* or occasionally *trans-acting factors.* (The prefix *trans* refers to the fact that these proteins may be encoded anywhere in the genome; the genes encoding transcription factors need not be physically linked to the genes they regulate.) Overall there appear to be hundreds of transcription factors, some of which interact with many genes, and some of which interact with only a small number of genes. Transcription factors can increase or decrease the rate of expression of the genes with which they interact, that is, they can act as transcriptional activators or repressors. As will be described later, some transcription factors activate genes only after they are modified by a physiological signal.

Given the large number of transcription factors and their differing functional properties, it is important that only the biologically appropriate factors be brought into proximity with the transcriptional start site of the genes they are meant to regulate. This is accomplished by individual transcription factors having specific binding sites on the DNA. Thus, they are tethered to their correct target genes, but not to other genes. The specificity of the binding site for a given protein is determined by the particular order of bases in that region of the DNA. The short stretches of DNA that bind transcription factors are called *cis*-regulatory elements (Figure 1–7). (The term *cis* indicates that they are contained on the same stretch of DNA as the genes they regulate.) By analogy with neuropharmacology, the specific DNA sequences of *cis*-regulatory elements can be thought of as receptors for transcription factors. In fact, the dissociation constants describing the binding affinities of these proteins for their DNA binding sites are in ranges quite similar to those of many drugs for neurotransmitter receptors.

In eukaryotes, multiple *cis*-regulatory elements are arrayed upstream (i.e., in the 5′ direction) (Figure 1–7), and occasionally downstream (i.e., in the 3′ direction), of the start site of transcription. Studies in which these sites have been mutated have shown that each gene has a particular combination of *cis*-regulatory elements, the nature, number, and spatial arrangement of which determine the gene's unique pattern of expression, including the cell types in which it is expressed, the times during development in which it is expressed, and the level at which it is expressed in adults both basally and in response to physiological signals.

Cis-regulatory elements are generally found within several hundred bases of the transcriptional start site, but can occasionally be found many thousands of base pairs away. The control region of a gene that is near the start site of transcription is called the *promoter*. Regulatory elements that exert control at some distance from the start site have been called *enhancers*, but this distinction appears to be artificial from a mechanistic point of view. Promoter and enhancer elements appear to function similarly; both are composed of smaller "modular" sequence elements (often 7–12 base pairs in length), each of which is a specific binding site for one or more transcription factors.

Much remains to be learned about the mechanism by which the proteins that bind to these elements regulate gene expression. Many such proteins contain two domains, one that recognizes and binds to a specific DNA sequence (i.e., to the *cis*-regulatory element) and a second domain that interacts with the transcription machinery (RNA polymerase II and associated proteins in the polymerase II transcription complex). The mechanism by which proteins binding to *cis*-regulatory elements far from the transcription start site can activate or repress transcription is not entirely clear, but the leading theory is that the DNA can loop out and thereby bring proteins bound to distant regions of the DNA into close contact with each other (Figure 1–8).

Many transcription factors are only active as dimers, either of identical proteins (homodimers) or of two different proteins (heterodimers). The ability of transcription factors to form heterodimers increases the diversity of transcription factor complexes that can form in cells and, as a result, increases the types of specific regulation that can be exerted on gene expression.

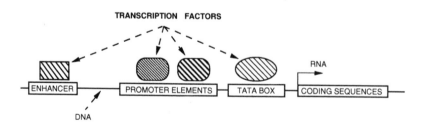

FIGURE 1–7. Schematic illustration of an idealized eukaryotic promoter. *Open rectangles* represent DNA regulatory elements that serve as binding sites for proteins *(hatched shapes)* involved in transcriptional regulation (see text for discussion). The protein that binds to the TATA box (TFIID) determines the exact start site of transcription.

Examples of regulatory mechanisms. Most eukaryotic promoters have a region rich in the nucleotides A and T located between 25 and 30 bases upstream of the transcription start site. This sequence, called a TATA box (Figure 1–7), binds a transcription factor called TFIID (polymerase II transcription factor D), which is required for exact positioning of the start site of transcription. If the TATA box is mutated, transcription initiation may not occur or may be inaccurate.

In addition to the TATA box, many promoters contain one or more *cis*-regulatory elements that bind transcription factors that confer a basal level of transcriptional activity on the gene. Many "basal" *cis*-regulatory elements are shared by many genes. Common examples are the GC box (rich in the nucleotides G and C), which binds a transcriptional activator protein called SP1, and the CCATT box, which binds several different transcription factors. A gene that contained these types of regulatory elements would be expressed constitutively (that is, at some finite level even when the cell is unstimulated), unless the gene also bound a repressor protein that prevented its expression under certain circumstances.

Because all cells of an organism contain the same DNA (i.e., a complete copy of the organism's genome), individual genes must contain regulatory elements that permit selective expression of the genes during development and adult life. Differential expression of a common genome is required for the formation of distinct cell types during development (e.g., neuron versus kidney versus liver cells), including the differentiation of thousands of distinct types of neurons

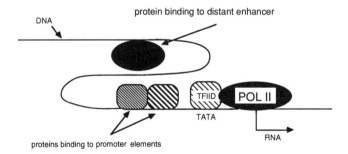

FIGURE 1–8. Hypothetical model to explain how proteins bound to enhancer elements far upstream of the transcription start site can regulate gene expression. According to this model, the DNA loops out and thereby brings all of the proteins bound to distant regions of the promoter in close proximity with RNA polymerase II (POL II) to form an active transcription complex. TFIID = polymerase II transcription factor D.

found in the brain. Differential gene expression also underlies the unique functional properties of these various cell types.

Differential gene expression is established by a number of mechanisms. Some genes contain *cis*-regulatory elements that bind transcriptional repressor proteins; the presence of the repressor proteins in a particular cell type would block expression of those genes in that cell type. (Presumably repressor proteins act by disrupting formation of an active polymerase II transcription complex.) Other genes may have their expression restricted to certain cell types if they lack *cis*-regulatory elements that bind ubiquitous transcriptional activators, but instead depend for their activation on proteins that themselves are found only in a limited number of cell types. This appears to be the case for the pituitary hormones growth hormone and prolactin. These are expressed only in pituitary lactotrophs and somatotrophs, the only adult cell types in which their main positive activator, a protein called Pit 1, is found. Of course, this leaves unanswered the question of how the selective expression of Pit 1 (a member of the POU family of transcription factors) is achieved.

In fact, mechanisms underlying the restriction of expression of genes only to appropriate cells comprise a complex subject that is understood in detail in only a few cases. It appears likely that specificity of gene expression is often achieved through a combination of mechanisms: a given gene may contain multiple types of both repressor binding sites and activator binding sites that act in concert to determine which cells can express that gene. It can be seen from this brief discussion that a major problem in developmental biology is understanding how cells come to express the particular set of activator and repressor proteins that determine which other genes will be expressed in that cell.

In addition to both ubiquitous and cell-type–specific (also called tissue-specific) *cis*-regulatory elements, many and possibly most genes contain *cis*-regulatory elements that bind proteins that activate transcription in response to a physiological signal. In the jargon of the field, elements that bind such proteins are often called "response elements" because they mediate regulation of gene expression in response to a particular physiological stimulus. One important family of physiologically regulated elements is the glucocorticoid response elements (GREs). Glucocorticoids bind to and thereby activate specific receptors within the cytoplasm of cells. The activated receptors then translocate into the nucleus, where they bind to GREs contained within particular genes. Such binding then increases or decreases the rate at which these target genes are transcribed, depending on the precise nature and DNA sequence context of the GRE. Most of the known effects of glucocorticoids on cell function are mediated via their regulation of gene expression. Very similar mechanisms are involved in mediating the effects on cell function of gonadal steroids, thyroid hormone, and vitamin D.

Another important type of response element is the *cyclic adenosine mono-phosphate (AMP) response element* (CRE), defined as a nucleotide sequence that confers cyclic AMP responsiveness on a gene. The major species of CRE appears to be the nucleotide sequence TGACGTCA or closely related sequences. This was determined by examining the promoter regions of a large number of genes known to exhibit cyclic AMP responsiveness. Extremely similar sequences, designated the CRE, were then identified within these genes. (Similar DNA sequences that confer a specific functional property can be referred to as *consensus sequences*.) The family of transcription factors that bind to CREs and thereby mediate the effects of cyclic AMP on gene expression have been termed *CRE binding proteins* or *CREB proteins*. Gene transcription is activated when CREB proteins are bound to their recognition sequence (i.e., the CRE) and are then phosphorylated by cyclic AMP–dependent protein kinase. As will be seen in Chapter 4, this is a mechanism by which the many neurotransmitters and drugs that regulate cyclic AMP levels within neurons may exert important effects on gene expression.

Another physiologically important response element confers activation of a gene in response to the protein kinase C signal transduction pathway. This element, with the consensus sequence TGACTCA, differs by only one base from the CRE consensus sequence, but binds a different set of proteins with different signal transduction properties. Because this element was first shown to bind a crude protein extract called activator protein-1 (AP-1), it is termed the *AP-1 site*. In recent years, the individual protein components of the AP-1 complex have been analyzed. For example, two of the main transcription factors found in the AP-1 complex are c-Fos and c-Jun, which bind to the AP-1 site when they combine as heterodimers.

As will be seen, many environmental signals regulate gene expression by activating biochemical cascades that lead to the activation of protein kinases and subsequently to the phosphorylation of specific transcription factors. One of the best understood examples is phosphorylation of CREB proteins by cyclic AMP–dependent protein kinase as mentioned above. However, many other types of transcription factors are also phosphorylated in response to environmental stimuli. The role played by transcription factor phosphorylation in the regulation of gene expression, and its potential importance to psychiatry, is discussed in detail in Chapter 4.

Processing RNA Into mRNA

Eukaryotic cells have far more DNA than is needed for genes. In human cells it appears that only about 1% of the DNA (comprising about 100,000 genes) encodes proteins that are actually made by the organism. Interestingly, beyond the minimum amount needed for genes, the total amount of DNA in the cells of a particular organism is unrelated to the complexity of that organism. Certain plants, for example, have more than 10 times as much DNA within their cells as is found in human cells. Much of the extra DNA in all eukaryotic organisms does not appear to code anything and much is composed of short repetitive sequence elements, often organized in long tandem arrays. (As will be seen in Chapter 6, these tandem repeats can be useful markers in human genetic analyses.) This extra DNA may serve some unknown function, such as a structural function for the nucleus. However, some have hypothesized that this extra DNA is parasitic: contributing nothing to the cell, but being replicated along with the cell's functional DNA.

It was initially a great surprise to geneticists that in eukaryotic cells "extra" DNA is found not only between genes, but within them. Whereas in bacteria, proteins are almost invariably encoded by a single uninterrupted stretch of DNA, in eukaryotes most genes have their coding sequences (called *exons*) interrupted by noncoding sequences (called *introns*). When a gene is transcribed, a long RNA is produced that is colinear with the DNA and therefore contains both exons and introns. This is called the *primary transcript.* Before this RNA leaves the nucleus, the introns are removed by RNA processing enzymes and the exons are joined to form a mature mRNA. This process is called *RNA splicing* (Figure 1–9) and is mediated by macromolecular RNA-protein complexes termed *spliceosomes.* (The term *exon* is derived from the fact that these sequences of DNA are *ex*ported, in the form of mRNA, from the nucleus.) Once splicing is completed, the mRNA leaves the nucleus and binds to a ribosome in the cytoplasm where it can direct the synthesis of a protein.

The process of splicing seems wasteful, but it may have evolved to increase the numbers of individual proteins than can be synthesized from a finite number of genes. In some cases, primary transcripts may be spliced in alternative ways, depending on the cell type or the stage of development, to produce a different mRNA and hence a different protein. This mechanism is used, for example, by cells within the nervous and endocrine systems to form two proteins—calcitonin in the thyroid gland to serve as a hormone, or calcitonin gene–related peptide in neurons to serve as a neurotransmitter—from the same primary transcript depending on which exons are retained or spliced out.

The existence of introns may also facilitate the genetic recombination of exons and may thus speed up the process by which new proteins can evolve from existing ones. This process of genetic recombination is thought to have been a powerful force through evolution of the species. One theory is that many individual exons code for functional domains of proteins (e.g., a catalytic site or a

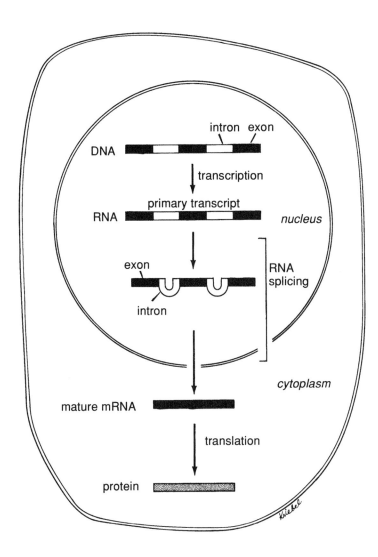

FIGURE 1–9.   Schematic illustration of RNA splicing. DNA contains both exons, which encode polypeptides, and introns, which do not. The primary RNA transcript produced by RNA polymerase II contains both exons and introns. Before the transcript leaves the nucleus, a series of enzymes (themselves partly composed of RNA) recognize particular sequences as exon-intron boundaries and splice out the intron sequences. The mature mRNA, containing only exons, is then exported from the nucleus into the cytoplasm, where it can bind to ribosomes and be translated into protein.

ligand recognition domain); the fact that they are separated by noncoding introns increases the likelihood that, during recombination or gene rearrangement events, the sequences coding functional domains would be preserved (i.e., the break would occur in an intron) and could remain functional when juxtaposed in novel ways to form new proteins with novel types of functions.

Translation of mRNA Into Protein

The rules governing the translation of mRNA into protein are called the *genetic code*. The sequence of nucleotides in the mRNA are "read" on ribosomes in serial order in groups of three. Each triplet of nucleotides specifies one amino acid and is called a *codon*. Because RNA is a linear polymer of four nucleotides, there are 64 (4^3) possible codons, but only 20 amino acids. As a result, although each codon specifies only a single amino acid, most amino acids are specified by more than one codon. The genetic code is therefore said to be *degenerate*. With only a few minor exceptions, the genetic code has been conserved across evolution.

Each mRNA sequence could potentially be read in any one of three different reading frames, depending on the nucleotide with which translation begins. In fact, there are specific initiator codons and stop codons that mark the beginning and end of translation and thereby set the correct reading frame. mRNAs also contain nucleotides before the start codon (5' untranslated sequences) and after the stop codon (3' untranslated sequences). Within the 3' untranslated region of most eukaryotic mRNAs are sequences recognized by enzymes that add long stretches of the nucleotide A [poly(A)] to the 3' end of the mRNA. The functional roles of untranslated regions and of the poly(A) tail of mRNAs are not fully understood, but may determine the relative "translatability" of the mRNA (i.e., the rate at which the message is translated into protein) and the relative stability of the mRNA (i.e., the rate at which it is degraded by RNase enzymes). Factors that influence the translatability or stability of an mRNA would alter the total amount of protein synthesized from that mRNA and could thereby play an important role in the regulation of cell function.

The codons in an mRNA molecule do not interact directly with the amino acids they specify; the translation of mRNA into protein depends on the presence of adaptor molecules that carry a particular amino acid and recognize the corresponding codon. These adaptors consist of a set of specific tRNAs. The salient feature of a tRNA is that it folds in such a way as to form 1) a covalent attachment for a specific amino acid, and 2) a loop of RNA with a sequence complementary to a particular codon (see Figure 1–10). This loop is called an *anticodon* and allows the tRNA to interact with the mRNA and to deliver its amino acid to the growing peptide chain. There is a specific tRNA for each amino acid–specifying codon.

The ribosome is a structure composed both of proteins and structural RNAs; these organelles provide a structure on which tRNAs can interact (via their anti-codons) with the codons of an mRNA in sequential order. The ribosome finds a specific start site on the mRNA that sets the reading frame and then moves along the mRNA molecule translating the nucleotide sequence one codon at a time, using tRNAs to add amino acids to the growing end of the polypeptide chain. Translation of mRNA into protein occurs from the 5′ to 3′ direction along the mRNA. The 5′ end of mRNA corresponds to the amino terminus of the protein, whereas the 3′ end corresponds to the carboxy terminus of the protein. When

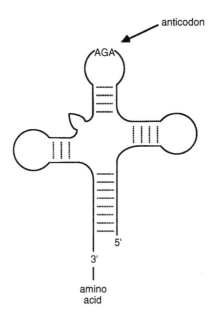

FIGURE 1–10. Chemical structure of tRNA. tRNA is a single strand of RNA that folds on itself through the apposition of complementary base pairs and the subsequent formation of hydrogen bonds, indicated by *dotted lines* in the figure. One of the loops formed contains the anticodon, the sequence of three nucleotides on the tRNA that binds to the complementary codon on an mRNA molecule. For the anticodon AGA shown in the figure, the corresponding codon on the mRNA would be UCU. The free 3′ end of the tRNA binds to a specific amino acid. Each tRNA, with a given anticodon, binds only one type of amino acid determined by the genetic code. In the case shown in the figure, the amino acid bound would be serine.

the ribosome reaches the end of the message, both the mRNA and the newly synthesized protein are released from the ribosome into the cytoplasm, and the ribosome dissociates into subunits. This process is illustrated schematically in Figure 1–11.

Posttranslational Regulation of Proteins

The amino acids of newly synthesized proteins may be chemically modified in a number of ways once they are released from the ribosome. There are enzymes that recognize certain consensus sequences of amino acids and add various chemical groups to particular amino acid residues within these recognition sequences. This is called *covalent modification* of proteins, because the proteins are altered by the formation of new chemical bonds. Addition of sugar groups to proteins is termed *glycosylation,* addition of phosphate groups *phosphorylation,* addition of acyl groups *acylation,* and so on.

Newly synthesized polypeptide chains also assume a particular three-dimensional conformation determined by their amino acid sequence and by these chemical modifications. A particular conformation can be determined by a number of factors, including the ability of certain amino acid side chains (those of

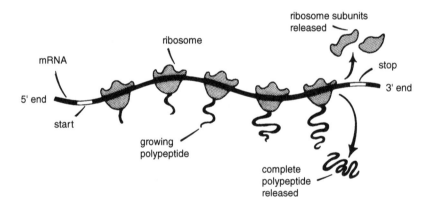

FIGURE 1–11. Schematic illustration of the translation of mRNA into protein. Ribosomal subunits bind together on mature mRNAs to form actively translating ribosomes. The ribosome begins adding amino acids when it reaches a start codon on the mRNA and processes down the mRNA, one codon at a time, adding the appropriate amino acid as it is delivered by a tRNA. When a stop codon is reached, the ribosome releases the polypeptide chain and dissociates from the mRNA. Each mRNA that is being actively translated has multiple ribosomes moving sequentially down its length, forming a polyribosome complex.

cysteine) to covalently bind to each other (so-called disulfide bonds), the ability of other amino acid side chains to form hydrogen bonds with each other, the relative hydrophobicity of particular side chains, the negative or positive charges on side chains, and the relative inflexibility of certain amino acids to bend or fold. Soluble proteins usually contain hydrophilic residues on the surface of their three-dimensional structures, with hydrophobic residues buried in their center. Proteins that span the plasma membrane (e.g., receptors) usually contain hydrophilic residues on the portions of the molecule exposed to the extracellular or intracellular milieu, with the transmembrane domains consisting of hydrophobic residues that anchor the proteins in the membrane lipid bilayer where they have no contact with water molecules. The three-dimensional conformation of a protein is a critical determinant of its function. For example, an ion channel protein must have a shape that permits it to be inserted into and to traverse the neuronal membrane, to have a pore that will admit only the correct ions, and to have a gating mechanism that allows the pore to open or close depending on the state of a cell.

In addition to covalent modification, proteins are subject to *allosteric regulation,* whereby their function is altered by a noncovalent (no chemical bond is formed) binding interaction with another molecule, often a small molecule. In allosteric interactions, the binding of a small molecule causes the protein to change its conformation and hence its functional activity. For example, many enzymes are allosterically regulated by nonprotein cofactors that bind to the enzymes and thereby increase or decrease their affinity for a particular substrate. The ability of a receptor to be functionally activated by hormone binding is another example of allosteric regulation.

Individual proteins can also bind to each other noncovalently to form multisubunit complexes (quaternary structure). The binding of proteins to one another is determined by their affinity for each other, which, in turn, is determined by their size, shape, and charge. Individual protein subunits of a multisubunit complex may subserve different functions and thereby contribute to the overall functional activity of the complex. For example, cyclic AMP–dependent protein kinase is composed of two copies of each of two types of subunit: regulatory and catalytic. All of the necessary enzymatic activity of the protein complex resides in the catalytic subunit, whereas the cyclic AMP dependence of the complex resides entirely within the regulatory subunit (see Chapter 2).

The very large number of proteins in a cell, their chemical and structural diversity, their ability to form multisubunit complexes, and the numerous ways in which their function can be modulated covalently and allosterically underlie the functional versatility of proteins and their ability to perform virtually every aspect of cell function. It is the types of proteins expressed in a given neuron, as well as their levels of expression, that imbue neurons with their distinctive developmental, structural, and functional properties. In thinking about how neurons can undergo long-term changes in function (e.g., to store memories or to respond to environmental events or psychotropic drugs), it would appear that critical mechanisms involve alterations in the levels of specific neuronal proteins or in their functional state as determined by covalent or allosteric modifications. In subsequent chapters, it will become apparent that a major goal of psychiatry today is to identify proteins that subserve specific functions in the nervous system and to determine how alterations in these proteins may underlie the causes, expression, and treatment of neuropsychiatric disorders.

SELECTED REFERENCES

Crick FHC: The genetic code: III. Sci Am 215:55–62, 1978
Maniatis T, Goodbourn S, Fischer JA: Regulation of inducible and tissue-specific gene expression. Science 236:1237–1245, 1987
Mitchell PJ, Tjian R: Transcriptional regulation in mammalian cells by sequence-specific DNA binding proteins. Science 245:371–378, 1989
Ptashne M: How gene activators work. Sci Am 261:41–47, 1989
Watson JD, Crick FHC: Molecular structure of nucleic acids: a structure for deoxyribose ´nucleic acid. Nature 171:964–967, 1953
Watson JD, Hopkins NH, Roberts JW, et al: Molecular Biology of the Gene, 4th Edition. Menlo Park, CA, Benjamin/Cummings, 1987

Chapter 2

Overview of

Synaptic

Neurotransmission

The brain receives, processes, and interprets multiple types of sensory stimuli; controls motor output; records experiences in the form of memory; carries out complicated cognitive tasks, including understanding and producing language; and is responsible for moods, for behavior, and, indeed, for consciousness itself. The brain is so extraordinarily complex that the mechanisms by which it functions have frequently been declared unknowable by mystics and obscurantists. The brain, however, is an organ, and like any organ it is composed of cells. All of the brain's functions are carried out by nerve cells (neurons) that communicate with each other in networks of remarkably complex but precise connections. In addition to neurons, the brain contains cells called glia that perform many important functions. This book, however, focuses almost exclusively on neurons, because, although glial cells are extremely interesting in their own right, they are not thought to play a primary role in information processing. Rather, they likely play a more supportive and permissive role in neuronal function.

A very crude estimate of the complexity of the human brain is to state that it contains approximately 100 billion neurons, among which there are perhaps tens of thousands of distinct neuronal cell types, each with different structural and functional properties. However, this approximation actually underestimates the

---

Text defined by vertical rules in the left margin involves advanced concepts and can be skipped by readers interested in a more general overview of the field, without loss of the overall message of the book.

complexity of the brain because the primary elements of information processing may not be neurons, but rather the individual connections that they make with each other, called *synapses*. At synapses (which are specialized gaps between neurons), neurons communicate with each other by releasing a chemical substance called a *neurotransmitter* that binds to and activates specific receptors on the neighboring neuron. Neurons in the brain can form a thousand, sometimes more than several thousand, synapses with other neurons. There are therefore likely to be more than 100 trillion synapses in a single human brain. Finally, neurons may release more than one neurotransmitter at any given synapse, adding yet another layer of complexity. Despite these staggering numbers, the study of the brain is not only possible, but is proceeding at an impressive rate. This chapter introduces the functions of neurons and the mechanisms by which they communicate with each other.

NEURONS

Neurons are irregularly shaped cells that possess three identifiable parts: a cell body, or soma, that gives rise to two types of processes—*dendrites* and *axons* (Figure 2–1). Most neurons give rise to multiple dendritic processes, which tend to be short and highly branched. Although there are exceptions, dendrites are generally the structure at which neurons receive incoming communications from other neurons; their primary receptive zones are often localized on specialized spines that protrude from the dendrite itself. In contrast, neurons usually give rise to a smaller number of axons, usually only one, that can be as long as the length of the entire organism. Axons typically branch at their ends to form

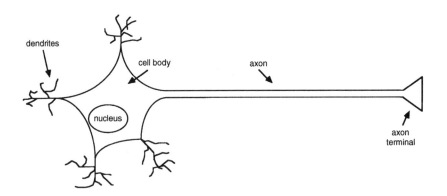

FIGURE 2–1. Schematic illustration of a neuron.

numerous projections that end in highly specialized structures called *axon terminals.* In most cases, axons and their terminals relay a neuron's output to other neurons.

Neurons are electrically excitable cells. This property, which is what allows neurons to process information and to communicate with each other, is based on the separation of ions (and therefore charge) by neuronal membranes, combined with mechanisms that selectively permit the flow of ions across the membrane under certain circumstances. The lipid bilayer that makes up the neuronal membrane is itself impermeable to ions, but contains within it several transporter proteins or "ion pumps" and a variety of ion channels (pores through which ions can passively diffuse). Neuronal ion channels are selective as to which ions can pass through and are tightly regulated or "gated." The ion pumps within neuronal membranes expend energy to keep the inside of the cell negatively charged with respect to the outside of the cell, that is, the neuronal membrane is electrically polarized. The degree of polarization in a quiescent neuron is called the *resting potential.*

Certain neurotransmitter receptors contain intrinsic ion channels in addition to their neurotransmitter recognition site. Neurotransmitter receptors that allow the entry of positively charged ions (cations) into neurons on stimulation (e.g., nicotinic acetylcholine receptors) make the local membrane potential less negative with respect to the outside; that is, they produce a *depolarization* of the membrane. Neurotransmitters that cause depolarization are, by definition, excitatory, because they bring a neuron toward its threshold for firing an *action potential.* Depending on the type of neurotransmitter and the type of receptor present on the neuron, the depolarization caused by an excitatory neurotransmitter can be large or small.

Inhibitory neurotransmitters cause *hyperpolarization* of the membrane, generally by admitting anions (making the inside of the neuron more negative with respect to the outside). Local depolarizations or hyperpolarizations resulting from neurotransmitter receptor activation occurring within dendrites or other parts of the neuron are called *synaptic potentials.* Synaptic potentials decrease in amplitude as they spread within the cell because they are dissipated by the passive electrical properties of the neuron, such as membrane capacitance.

When the balance between excitatory and inhibitory synaptic potentials produces a threshold degree of depolarization within the neuron, and more particularly within the initial segment of the neuron's axon, an action potential is produced within the axon. The action potential travels down the axon and ultimately depolarizes the plasma membrane of its presynaptic terminals. Depolarization of the axon terminal permits release of neurotransmitter and, therefore, communication with the next neuron in the circuit. In contrast to synaptic potentials, which are local signals, action potentials are self-renewing and propagate without fail down the length of the axon. Although signal processing and propagation of signals within neurons are critically dependent on ionic currents, communication between neurons is almost always carried by chemical rather than electrical signals. The mechanisms by which neuronal communication occurs will now be described in more detail.

Ionic Basis of Synaptic Transmission

Like all cells, neurons have external plasma membranes that separate their cytoplasmic components from the extracellular space. Plasma membranes are *semipermeable,* which means that only some substances can move freely across the membrane; most substances, including most ions, are impermeant and can only move across the membrane via specific protein channels or carriers (e.g., ion channels, transporters, and pumps).

Neurons use their plasma membranes, and the regulation of ion flow across the membrane, to establish an electrical potential difference between the intracellular and extracellular space. The concentration of Na^+ is high extracellularly, where it is the major extracellular cation (positively charged ion). K^+ has the opposite distribution; it is the major intracellular cation. Cl^- is the major extracellular anion (negatively charged ion); it is largely balanced intracellularly by negatively charged amino acids. The divalent cations Ca^{2+} and Mg^{2+}, like Na^+, are present in the extracellular fluid at much higher concentrations than intracellularly, but their extracellular concentrations are far lower than that of Na^+ (Figure 2–2).

Control of the distribution of ions across neuronal plasma membranes, and thus the regulation of electrical charge across the membrane (termed the *membrane potential*), is the critical mechanism underlying neuronal activity. The uneven distribution of anions and cations across the plasma membrane produces a resting potential of about -70 mV compared with the outside in an average neuron. As discussed above, appropriate stimuli can cause the membrane to depolarize or hyperpolarize. When a depolarization reaches a critical threshold (usually about -40 mV) in the initial segment of a neuron's axon (called the *trigger zone*), an action potential is generated whereby a rapid wave of depolarization passes down the axon and, without fail, propagates to the axon's terminals. This is followed by rapid repolarization of the axonal and terminal membrane, which reestablishes the original membrane potential. This process normally occurs within a few milliseconds.

Based on the pioneering studies of Hodgkin and Huxley, we know that action potentials are mediated through specific voltage-dependent Na^+ and K^+ chan-

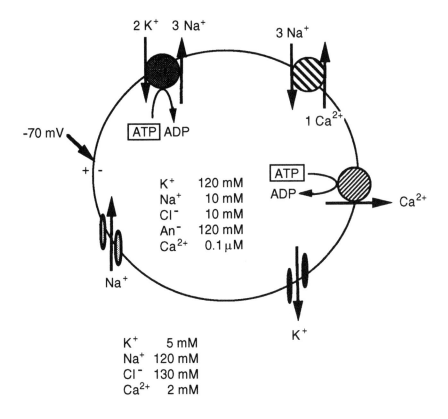

FIGURE 2–2. Schematic illustration of a neuronal cell showing ion concentrations and ion pumps. The concentrations of intracellular and extracellular ions are shown in millimoles per liter. These ion gradients result in a resting membrane potential of approximately −70 mV.

Also shown are three of the important transport proteins found in neuronal membranes. The Na^+-K^+ ATPase exchanges 2 K^+ ions for 3 Na^+ ions. Because this transporter is pumping ions against their electrochemical driving force, it uses energy in the form of ATP. Na^+-K^+ ATPase is one of the key actors in maintaining the resting potential. Two other transporters that serve to keep intracellular Ca^{2+} levels low are shown. One of these is dependent on ATP; the other uses the energy from allowing 3 Na^+ ions into the cell to pump out 1 Ca^{2+} ion against its electrochemical gradient. The resting intracellular concentration of Ca^{2+} is extremely low; in higher concentrations it not only functions as a cation to depolarize neurons, but also has important second messenger functions.

Also shown are the voltage-gated Na^+ and K^+ channels that are responsible for the depolarization and repolarization of the neuron during the action potential.

nels present in neuronal plasma membranes. Such ion channels are proteins that form pores in the membrane through which the specific types of ion can pass. The size and electrical properties of the pore determine the selectivity of a given channel for a particular ion. Under resting conditions, the ion channels are closed and the ions cannot move across the membrane. When a neuron's membrane potential is depolarized to a critical threshold, the change in voltage activates these channels—that is, they open, permitting the passive movement of ions down their electrochemical gradient. Because it is the membrane potential that controls or "gates" the opening of these channels, they are called *voltage-gated ion channels*. When voltage-gated Na^+ channels are open, Na^+ will enter from the outside of the neuron because there is a net electrochemical driving force on Na^+ ions in the inward direction: the concentration of Na^+ is higher in the extracellular space and the interior of the neuron is relatively negatively charged. In contrast, the net driving force on K^+ ions is outward because the concentration of K^+ is higher intracellularly than extracellularly.

Action potentials result from the successive opening and closing of Na^+ and K^+ channels in response to an adequate depolarizing stimulus. With a threshold depolarization, voltage-gated Na^+ channels rapidly open; this leads, in turn, to a further depolarization of the membrane. The threshold for generation of an action potential is the membrane potential at which a critical mass of Na^+ channels are open. This leads to complete depolarization of the membrane. The action potential propagates without fail because the depolarization of each segment of the neuronal membrane then brings its neighboring segment to threshold for opening of Na^+ channels, and so on. Because the opening of some Na^+ channels recruits additional channels into the process, they reinforce the depolarization within each axon segment, rather than allowing it to dissipate. This mechanism allows extremely rapid conduction of impulses over long distances, for example, in axons that run from the spinal cord to the tip of one's toe.

The action potential is terminated by two processes that occur in response to membrane depolarization a short time after the opening of voltage-gated Na^+ channels. The Na^+ channels close with a stereotyped time course after their opening and for a time are inactivated. In addition, voltage-gated K^+ channels are also caused to open by the passing depolarization, but their latency to opening is slower than that for Na^+ channels. Thus, after a lag, K^+ channels open and allow positive charges to exit the neuron, resulting in a wave of repolarization of the membrane. This series of rapid ionic events—Na^+ channel opening followed by Na^+ channel inactivation and K^+ channel opening—occurs in milliseconds and produces a discrete wave of depolarization that sweeps across the neuronal membrane and passes down the length of the axon. After an action potential, the baseline concentrations of Na^+ and K^+ across the membrane are reestablished, much more slowly, via the Na^+-K^+ ATPase pump, which transfers Na^+ out of the cell and K^+ into the cell in a process that requires energy in the form of adenosine triphosphate (ATP).

Depolarization of the axon terminals results in the opening of voltage-dependent Ca^{2+} channels in the terminal membrane, and this leads to the flow of Ca^{2+} into the terminals. As first demonstrated by Katz and his colleagues, increased levels of Ca^{2+} within the terminals directly trigger the release of neurotransmitter into the synaptic cleft. The released neurotransmitter then acts on (e.g., produces synaptic potentials in) the postsynaptic neuron to alter its electrical properties, and so on.

In reality, the regulation of neuronal membrane excitability is far more complicated than described above. First, neuronal plasma membranes exhibit a great diversity of ion channel proteins that display different cellular distributions and functional activities. There are numerous types of voltage-dependent Na^+, K^+, and Ca^{2+} channels, as well as voltage-dependent channels for other ions. In addition, there are ion channels that are not voltage dependent, for example, ion channels that open or close in response to other ions (i.e., ion-gated ion channels such as Ca^{2+}-dependent K^+ channels) or ion channels that exist as part of a neurotransmitter receptor complex and are activated as a direct result of neurotransmitter receptor binding (i.e., ligand-gated ion channels, such as the nicotinic acetylcholine receptor, discussed later in this chapter). Molecular biological studies continue to reveal an increasing number and diversity of ion channels.

Second, the functional activity of many types of ion channels can be modulated by various stimuli. For example, in addition to simply determining whether ion channels are in an "opened" or "closed" state, stimuli can alter the response properties of ion channels over long periods. These types of modulatory processes will be discussed further in Chapter 3.

Synaptic Organization of the Brain

As described above, neurons communicate with one another at synapses. Most neurons communicate via chemical synapses. At a chemical synapse (Figure 2–3), the depolarization of a presynaptic axon terminal causes the release of a chemical substance, termed *neurotransmitter,* from the terminal. The neurotransmitter then diffuses across the synapse and binds to specialized receptor proteins on the postsynaptic dendrite or cell body. The binding of neurotransmitter to the receptor then establishes electrical changes in that postsynaptic cell that can be communicated in turn to other neurons. Neurotransmitter receptor

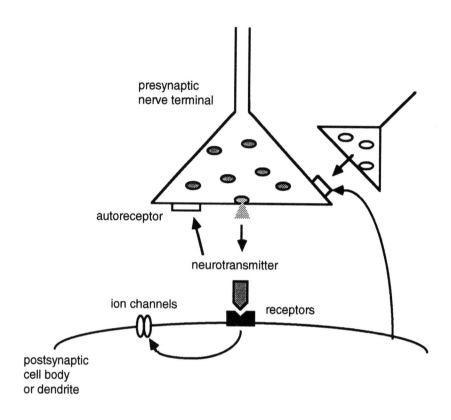

FIGURE 2–3.   Schematic illustration of synaptic transmission. Synaptic transmission involves the release of neurotransmitter, stored in synaptic vesicles, from a presynaptic nerve terminal; the neurotransmitter diffuses across the synaptic cleft and then binds to receptors on postsynaptic cell bodies or dendrites, leading to a change in ion channel conductances. This type of synapse is termed an *axosomatic* or *axodendritic* synapse in that it involves an axon terminal innervating a cell body (i.e., soma) or dendrite.

In addition, the figure illustrates that neurotransmitter receptors are also located on presynaptic nerve terminals. Some of these are *autoreceptors*—that is, they recognize the neurotransmitter released by that same nerve terminal. Others recognize neurotransmitter released by other nerve terminals (i.e., *axoaxonic synapses*, which are common in brain tissue), or, in a small number of cases, neurotransmitter released by dendrites (i.e., *dendroaxonic synapses*).

activation also leads to many other types of physiological responses in target neurons that will be described later in this chapter.

Different neuronal cell types in the brain utilize different neurotransmitters; between 50 and 100 different molecules are either proven neurotransmitters or convincing candidates for functioning as neurotransmitters. Similarly, neurons express different types of receptors for neurotransmitters, with most neurotransmitters able to interact with more than one type of receptor. The diversity of neurotransmitters and neurotransmitter receptors adds an important layer of complexity to the brain over and above its "wiring diagram."

The classical synapse (Figure 2–4, *A*) is termed *axodendritic* or *axosomatic* in that presynaptic axon terminals innervate postsynaptic dendrites or cell bodies. In recent years, it has become apparent that the synaptic organization of the brain is much more varied, such that the distinction between presynaptic and postsynaptic function can no longer be made entirely on the basis of anatomical criteria. Thus, many axon terminals in the brain are themselves functionally postsynaptic to other axon terminals. In this situation, the terminals possess receptors on their plasma membrane that respond to neurotransmitters released by neighboring axon terminals (Figure 2–4, *B*). This type of synaptic communication is referred to as *axoaxonic*. In addition, many, and possibly most, axon terminals possess receptors on their plasma membrane that respond to the neurotransmitter they release; these receptors are termed *autoreceptors* and serve as feedback mechanisms by which the amount of neurotransmitter released by a nerve terminal is regulated by preceding release events (Figure 2–4, *C*). In this sense, many axon terminals respond postsynaptically to their own neurotransmitter. Finally, in a small number of cases, neurotransmitter can even be released by certain dendrites in the brain. Neurotransmitters released from dendrites appear to bind to receptors on presynaptic nerve terminals, where they influence the release of neurotransmitter from those terminals (e.g., in the substantia nigra; Figure 2–4, *E*), or on other dendrites (e.g., in the retina; Figure 2–4, *D*). Such synapses are termed *dendroaxonic* and *dendrodendritic,* respectively.

It is probable that, for most neurons in the brain, a combination of synaptic connections exist. For example, as shown in Figure 2–4, *F,* neurotransmitter released from a nerve terminal would influence other nerve terminals and a population of cell bodies in its immediate vicinity. In addition, the function of that terminal would, in turn, be influenced by neurotransmitters released from other nerve terminals and dendrites.

Although transmission at most synapses in the brain is chemical (i.e., mediated by neurotransmitters), communication between some neurons is electrical. In this situation, a wave of depolarization travels from one neuronal process directly into a neighboring neuron via minute connections called *gap junctions*.

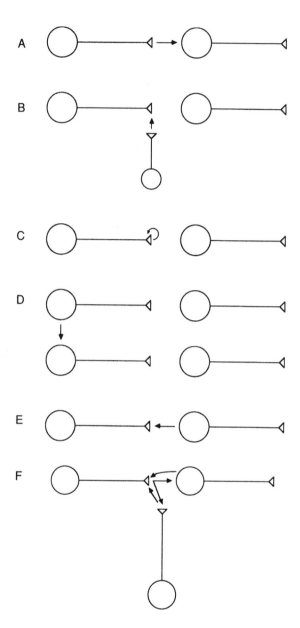

FIGURE 2–4. Synaptic organization of the brain. *A:* Axodendritic, or axosomatic, synapse. *B:* Axoaxonic synapse. *C:* Synapse with autoreceptor. *D:* Dendrodendritic synapse. *E:* Dendroaxonic synapse. *F:* Combination of synaptic connections. See text for discussion.   *Source.* Modified from Nestler EJ, Greengard P: *Protein Phosphorylation in the Nervous System.* New York, Wiley, 1984. Used with permission.

Such electrical synapses were thought to be extremely rare in the adult mammalian brain, but recent studies indicate that they may occur with greater frequency than previously believed.

NEUROTRANSMITTERS IN THE BRAIN

A neurotransmitter is defined as a chemical that is synthesized in a neuron, is released by that neuron in response to electrical impulses, and acts on other neurons to alter their electrical properties. Tables 2–1 and 2–2 list the types of molecules that mammalian neurons use as neurotransmitters.

The most prevalent neurotransmitters in the central nervous system (CNS) are the excitatory amino acid glutamate (and possibly aspartate) and the inhibitory amino acids γ-aminobutyric acid (GABA) and glycine. It has been estimated that these amino acids are utilized as neurotransmitters by 75%–90% of all of the neurons in the brain and spinal cord.

Other neurotransmitters are present at far fewer synapses. The monoamine neurotransmitters are divided into two major classes based on chemical structure—the catecholamines and indoleamines. The catecholamines include dopamine, norepinephrine, and epinephrine, and the indoleamines include serotonin and melatonin. Acetylcholine, the major neurotransmitter at the mammalian neuromuscular junction, also plays an important role as a neurotransmitter in the

TABLE 2–1. Neurotransmitters in the brain

Amino acids	
Excitatory	Glutamate
	?Aspartate
Inhibitory	GABA
	Glycine
Monoamines	
Catecholamines	Dopamine
	Norepinephrine
	Epinephrine
Indoleamines	Serotonin
	Melatonin
Other	Histamine
Acetylcholine	
Others	Nitric oxide
	Purines (e.g., adenosine)

Note. GABA = γ-aminobutyric acid.

brain. In addition, neurotransmitter functions for histamine (also a monoamine), purines (e.g., adenosine), and nitric oxide have been proposed.

In addition to these small molecules, it is now known that a number of peptides function as neurotransmitters. The exact number of neuropeptides believed to function in this capacity is continually growing; a partial list is shown in Table 2–2. Neuropeptides can be organized into a number of general categories. For example, peptides used by hypothalamic neurons to regulate release of hormones from the anterior pituitary are also used by hypothalamic and other neurons in the brain as neurotransmitters to mediate some of the synaptic actions of those neurons on other target neurons. As another example, a number of "gut" peptides that were identified originally in the gastrointestinal tract, where they regulate digestive processes, are also present in brain neurons, where they function as neurotransmitters. Still another example are the peptides derived from the common precursor pro-opiomelanocortin; these include adrenocorticotropic hormone (ACTH), α-melanocyte–stimulating hormone (α-MSH), and β-endorphin. A related group is the enkephalins, which are opioid peptides structurally related to the endorphins but derived from a distinct precursor pro-enkephalin. Each of these various peptides appears to serve neurotransmitter roles for specific populations of neurons in the CNS.

Small-molecule neurotransmitters are synthesized by enzymatic pathways. Neuropeptides, like all proteins, are synthesized by transcription of genes and

---

TABLE 2–2.   Neuropeptides

Opioid and related peptides
  Endorphins
  Enkephalins
  Adrenocorticotropic hormone
    (ACTH)
  Melanocyte-stimulating
    hormone (MSH)

Gut-brain peptides
  Vasoactive intestinal polypeptide
    (VIP)
  Cholecystokinin (CCK)
  Secretin
  Somatostatin
  Neuropeptide Y

Tachykinin peptides
  Substance P
  Substance K
  Neuromedin

Posterior pituitary peptides
  Oxytocin
  Vasopressin

Hypothalamic releasing factors
  Corticotropin-releasing factor
    (CRF)
  Thyrotropin-releasing factor (TRF)
  Growth hormone–releasing factor
    (GHRF)
  Luteinizing hormone–releasing
    factor (LHRH)

Others
  Calcitonin gene–related peptide
  Angiotensin
  Neurotensin

---

translation of the resulting messenger RNA (mRNA). Neuropeptides are produced as larger precursor proteins that are then enzymatically cleaved and modified to produce active neurotransmitter.

Neurotransmitters are synthesized in cell bodies of neurons and then packaged into vesicles and transported down axons into axon terminals, where they are stored for release. The brain contains synaptic vesicles of different sizes and staining properties (e.g., small versus large and clear versus dense-core vesicles) that appear to contain different types of neurotransmitter substances. In the case of small-molecule neurotransmitters, synthetic enzymes may be transported down the axon to the terminal; this allows the synthesis of the neurotransmitter locally in the axon terminals, in addition to cell bodies. In response to depolarization of the axon terminal plasma membrane, neurotransmitter is released by exocytosis, a Ca^{2+}-triggered process in which vesicles stored in the nerve terminals are transported to the terminal plasma membrane surface, fuse with the membrane, and release their contents into the synaptic cleft (see Figure 2–3). The exact molecular mechanisms underlying exocytosis and vesicle traffic within nerve terminals are a subject of great current interest. Released neurotransmitter then binds to presynaptic and postsynaptic receptors. The action of neurotransmitter in the synapse is terminated either by enzymatic degradation or, for some types of neurotransmitters, such as the monoamines, by transport back into the nerve terminals, where it is repackaged into vesicles and prepared for subsequent release events.

Colocalization of Neurotransmitters in the Brain

It has become apparent in recent years that individual neurons frequently utilize more than one neurotransmitter for synaptic transmission. This finding contradicts what had been called Dale's law: one neuron, one transmitter. Indeed, multiple transmitters within a single neuron may be the rule rather than the exception in the CNS, and even to some extent in the periphery. In most cases, neurons contain an amino acid, a monoamine, or acetylcholine plus one or more neuropeptides; some examples are given in Table 2–3. For example, certain neurons of the locus coeruleus contain not only norepinephrine, but also enkephalin, somatostatin, and/or neuropeptide Y. A subset of peripheral parasympathetic neurons contain vasoactive intestinal polypeptide (VIP) as well as acetylcholine, and peripheral sympathetic neurons may contain neuropeptide Y as well as norepinephrine.

Peptides and small-molecule neurotransmitters coexisting within the same cells may be packaged in the same vesicles and released together. This appears to be the case in the adrenal medulla for norepinephrine and enkephalin, as well as for several other peptides. More often, colocalized neurotransmitters are packaged in separate vesicles and released from the same nerve terminal under different conditions. This appears to be the case in some peripheral and central catecholaminergic neurons, where the catecholamine neurotransmitter is released with low-frequency firing, and both the catecholamine and its colocalized neuropeptide are released with higher-frequency firing. The function served by colocalization of neurotransmitters is unknown. Increasing evidence suggests that, at least in many cases, the peptide neurotransmitter may serve a modulatory role by modifying the main actions of the other neurotransmitter.

NEUROTRANSMITTER RECEPTORS IN THE BRAIN

Neurotransmitter receptors are proteins that mediate the actions of specific neurotransmitters on target neurons. They are found on the plasma membrane of dendrites, cell bodies, and/or axon terminals of neurons. Neurotransmitters bind to specific sites on receptor proteins. Such binding leads to alterations in the physical properties of the receptors that result in transduction of the extracellular signal (neurotransmitter binding) into an intracellular signal, which leads, in turn, to alterations in the functional state of the target neurons.

Before the availability of modern methods for identifying neurotransmitter receptors directly, their existence was inferred from pharmacological evidence. In particular, the very low concentrations at which many psychotropic drugs act in vivo suggested that they interact highly specifically with only a small number

TABLE 2–3. Examples of colocalization of neurotransmitters

Small-molecule neurotransmitter	Peptide neurotransmitter	Neurons showing colocalization
GABA	Enkephalin Substance P	Striatal neurons
Norepinephrine	Somatostatin Neuropeptide Y	Sympathetic neurons Locus coeruleus neurons
Dopamine	Cholecystokinin Neurotensin	Ventral tegmental neurons
Acetylcholine	VIP CGRP	Cortical, parasympathetic neurons Motor neurons
Serotonin	Substance P	Raphe neurons

Note. GABA = γ-aminobutyric acid. VIP = vasoactive intestinal polypeptide. CGRP = calcitonin gene–related peptide.

of target molecules. Similarly, the existence of competitive antagonists that also act at low concentrations to block the effects of a putative endogenous ligand or of exogenous agonists provided further evidence for specific receptors.

Since the early 1970s, neurotransmitter receptors have been identified and characterized primarily by studying the direct binding of radioactively labeled molecules to receptors in crude membrane fractions of brain tissue or in histological sections of brain. Such pharmacological analysis has led to the identification of multiple types of receptors for each neurotransmitter, some of which are shown in Table 2–4. Receptor types are defined pharmacologically by a reproducible rank order of potency by which they interact with various drugs. In terms of direct ligand binding methods this can be restated in terms of binding affinity: each receptor has a characteristic rank order of binding affinities for a set of drugs. For example, all adrenergic receptors bind many of the same compounds, but α_1-adrenergic receptors have a rank order of pharmacological potency and binding affinity of epinephrine $\geq$ norepinephrine $>>$ isoproterenol, whereas β_1-adrenergic receptors have the rank order of isoproterenol $>$ epinephrine = norepinephrine.

More recently, molecular biological techniques, in which individual receptor proteins are cloned and expressed in vitro, have not only indicated that the various pharmacological subtypes of receptors generally represent distinct proteins, but have also led to the identification of still larger numbers of receptor subtypes. For example, whereas two major subtypes of muscarinic cholinergic receptors, M_1 and M_2, have been identified by pharmacological analyses, at least four distinct protein products are known through cloning studies.

Work is now needed to determine which specific cloned receptor protein corresponds to the pharmacological subtypes identified earlier. Work is also needed to establish the precise differences in the anatomical and functional properties of the numerous receptor subtypes. It is likely that such heterogeneity in neurotransmitter receptors underlies the ways in which various neuronal cell types respond differently to the same neurotransmitters. Such receptor heterogeneity also offers the future possibility of developing compounds with increased specificity at particular receptor subtypes that would have the potential of being more effective and safer pharmacotherapeutic agents in neuropsychiatric disorders.

Neurotransmitter receptors can be divided into two major categories based on whether they influence the activity of ion channels directly or indirectly via biochemical intermediates (see Table 2–4). Some neurotransmitter receptor proteins contain an intrinsic membrane-spanning ion channel. These receptors transduce an extracellular signal (ligand binding) into an intracellular signal by opening their intrinsic channel; these are therefore termed *ligand-gated ion channels* or *receptor-ionophores* (Figure 2–5, *A*). Examples of ligand-gated channels include the nicotinic acetylcholine receptor, the GABA$_A$ receptor, most types of glutamate receptors, and the 5-HT$_3$ (serotonin) receptor. In contrast, most types of neurotransmitter receptors, including all of the adrenergic and dopamine receptors, do not contain ion channels within their structures. Because they produce their cellular effects by acting through intervening cellular trans-

TABLE 2–4. Neurotransmitter receptors reported in the brain

Neurotransmitter	Receptor subtype	G protein linked (G) vs. ligand-gated channel (LG)
Dopamine	D$_1$	G
	D$_2$	G
	D$_3$	G
	D$_4$	G
	D$_5$	G
Norepinephrine and epinephrine	α_1	G
	α_2	G
	β_1	G
	β_2	G
	β_3	G
Serotonin	5-HT$_{1a}$	G
	5-HT$_{1b}$	G
	5-HT$_{1c}$	G
	5-HT$_{1d}$	G
	5-HT$_2$	G
	5-HT$_3$	LG
Acetylcholine	muscarinic M$_1$	G
	muscarinic M$_2$	G
	muscarinic M$_3$	G
	muscarinic M$_4$	G
	nicotinic	LG
Endorphins and enkephalins	δ	G
	μ	G
	κ	G
Glutamate	NMDA	LG
	AMPA	LG
	kainate	LG
	metabotropic	G
GABA	A	LG
	B	G

Note. NMDA = *N*-methyl-D-aspartate. AMPA = α-amino-3-hydroxy-5-methyl-4-isoxalone propionic acid. GABA = γ-aminobutyric acid.

ducing proteins called G proteins (so named because of their ability to bind guanine nucleotides), and in some cases other intracellular messengers (see Figure 2–5, *B* and *C*), these receptors are called *G protein–linked receptors.*

Many neurotransmitter receptors of both types have been cloned and sequenced. The ligand-gated channels and the G protein–linked receptors have each been found to represent distinct gene "families" with high degrees of protein sequence similarity (i.e., homology) within each family, but not between the two. This is consistent with the idea that the ligand-gated channels and the G protein–linked receptors each evolved from single (but unrelated) primordial ancestors by processes of gene duplication and mutation. It is also likely that during evolution regions of DNA encoding neurotransmitter recognition sites and regions encoding effector domains (e.g., membrane-spanning channels or G protein–binding moieties) were swapped by processes of gene rearrangement, leading to the situation in which, for example, there are acetylcholine receptors that are ligand-gated channels (nicotinic receptors) and others that are G protein–linked (muscarinic receptors). A similar theme of evolutionary conservation has been found to hold true for a third distinct family of proteins, which comprise the voltage-gated and ion-gated ion channels described above.

Synaptic responses mediated by ligand-gated channels and G protein–linked receptors show different temporal characteristics. Those mediated by ligand-

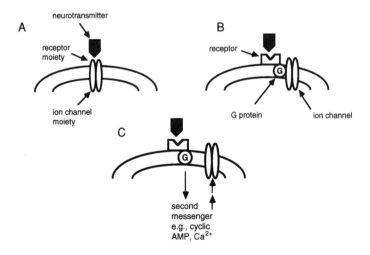

FIGURE 2–5.   Schematic illustration of the types of coupling of neurotransmitter receptors to ion channels. *A* shows a ligand-gated ion channel. *B* and *C* show G protein–linked receptors. See text for discussion.

gated channels are usually extremely rapid and short lived and are typically completed in less than 1 millisecond, whereas those mediated by G protein–linked receptors are generally slower in onset (requiring several milliseconds to seconds to develop) and can be very long in duration (up to many minutes).

The functional activity of neurotransmitter receptors can be modulated by a variety of stimuli. Thus, in addition to being in an "inactive" state (unbound to neurotransmitter) or an "activated" state (bound to neurotransmitter), various stimuli can alter the sensitivity of the receptor to its neurotransmitter (i.e., the ease with which the receptor is activated) and the ability of the receptor once activated to influence its effector, that is, an ion channel or other cellular process.

SIGNAL TRANSDUCTION IN THE BRAIN

Signal transduction refers to the processes by which binding of neurotransmitters to receptors, located on the extracellular aspect of the neuronal plasma membrane, produces alterations in neuronal functioning. Some of the pathways by which neurotransmitter-receptor interactions produce their diverse effects on target neurons are now well established and involve a complex network of intracellular messenger systems involving G proteins, second messengers, and protein phosphorylation. These pathways are summarized in Figure 2–6 and shown in more detail in Figures 2–8 and 2–9.

Intracellular messenger pathways can be viewed as subserving three major functions in the nervous system. First, they mediate certain short-term aspects of synaptic transmission: the rapid actions of neurotransmitters on ion channels other than those involving ligand-gated channels (i.e., all G protein–linked receptors) are achieved through intracellular messengers.

Second, intracellular messenger pathways play the central role in mediating other aspects of synaptic transmission: virtually all other actions of neurotransmitters on target neuron functioning, both short-term and long-term, are achieved through intracellular messengers (Figure 2–6). As will be seen in Chapter 4, these include those long-term actions of neurotransmitters that are mediated through alterations in neuronal gene expression. It is important to emphasize that such a role for intracellular messengers is not limited to actions of neurotransmitters mediated via G protein–linked receptors. Thus, although activation of ligand-gated ion channels leads to initial changes in electrical activity without the involvement of intracellular messengers, activation of these same receptors also leads to numerous additional (albeit slower) effects that are mediated via intracellular messengers.

Third, by virtue of numerous interactions among the various intracellular messenger pathways, these pathways play the central role in coordinating myriad neuronal processes and adjusting neuronal function to environmental cues.

G Proteins in Brain Signal Transduction Pathways

With the exception of synaptic transmission mediated via receptors that contain intrinsic ion channels, the family of membrane proteins known as G proteins may be involved in all other transmembrane signaling in the nervous system. G proteins, first identified and characterized by Rodbell, Gilman, and others, are so named because of their ability to bind the guanine nucleotides guanosine triphosphate (GTP) and guanosine diphosphate (GDP). G proteins serve to couple receptors to specific intracellular effector systems (Figure 2–6).

Three major types of G proteins are involved in transduction of signals produced by neurotransmitter binding: G_s, G_i, and G_o. Rhodopsin, the light-sensitive molecule of photoreceptor cells in the retina, can also be viewed as a G protein–linked receptor: light activates rhodopsin, which then, through a fourth type of G protein called transducin (G_t), regulates the electrical properties of photoreceptor cells. Each type of G protein is a heterotrimer composed of single α, β, and γ subunits. Distinct α subunits confer specific functional activity on the different types of G proteins, which appear to share common β and γ subunits.

The functional activity of G proteins is shown schematically in Figure 2–7. In the resting state, G proteins exist as heterotrimers that are bound to GDP and are unassociated with extracellular receptors or intracellular effector proteins (Figure 2–7, *A*). When the receptor is activated by ligand binding, a conformational change in the receptor causes its association with the α subunit of the G protein (Figure 2–7, *B*). This, in turn, alters the conformation of the α subunit and leads to 1) the exchange of GDP for GTP on the α subunit, 2) the dissociation of the β and γ subunits (which stay associated) from the α subunit, and 3) the release of the receptor from the G protein (Figure 2–7, *B* and *C*). This leads to the generation of free α subunit bound to GTP, which is biologically active and regulates the functional activity of effector proteins within the cell. There is also some evidence, albeit less definitive, that free β/γ subunits may also have biological activity. The system returns to its resting state when the ligand is released from the receptor and the GTPase activity that resides in the α subunit hydrolyzes GTP to GDP (Figure 2–7, *D*). The latter action leads to the reassociation of the free α subunit with the β/γ subunits to restore the original heterotrimers.

G protein regulation of ion channels.   G proteins have been shown to couple neurotransmitter receptors to multiple types of intracellular effector proteins. In some cases, G proteins couple neurotransmitter receptors directly to ion channels (Figure 2–7, C). Examples of this type of mechanism are the coupling of opiate, α_2-adrenergic, D_2 (dopaminergic), muscarinic cholinergic, 5-HT_{1a} (serotonergic), and $GABA_B$ receptors to a specific type of K^+ channel via subtypes of G_o and/or G_i in many types of neurons. Other types of ion channels may be similarly coupled to neurotransmitter receptors via G proteins.

G protein regulation of intracellular second messengers.   In many other cases, G proteins transduce the activation of neurotransmitter receptors (by neurotransmitter binding) into alterations in intracellular levels of second messengers in target neurons (see Figure 2–6). Prominent second messengers in the brain include cyclic AMP, cyclic guanosine monophosphate (GMP), Ca^{2+}, and the major metabolites of phosphatidylinositol (inositol triphosphate [IP_3] and diacylglycerol). As discussed above, altered levels of second mes-

FIGURE 2–6 *(at right).*   **Schematic illustration of the role played by intracellular messenger systems in synaptic transmission in the brain.** Recent studies in neuroscience have provided a considerably more complex view of synaptic transmission than that presented in Figure 2–3. These studies have focused on the involvement of intracellular messenger systems—involving coupling factors (termed G proteins), second messengers (e.g., cyclic AMP, cyclic GMP, Ca^{2+}, and the metabolites of phosphatidylinositol [PI]), and protein phosphorylation (involving the phosphorylation of phosphoproteins by protein kinases and their dephosphorylation by protein phosphatases)—in mediating multiple actions of neurotransmitters on their target neurons.

The figure illustrates three major roles subserved by these intracellular messengers. In some cases, intracellular messenger pathways mediate the actions of some neurotransmitters in opening or inhibiting particular ion channels. However, intracellular messengers mediate most of the many other actions of neurotransmitters on their target neurons. Some are relatively short lived and involve modulation of the general metabolic state of the neurons, their ability to synthesize or release neurotransmitter, and the functional sensitivity of their various receptors and ion channels to various synaptic inputs. Others are relatively long lived and are achieved through the regulation of gene expression in the target neurons. Thus, neurotransmitters, through the regulation of intracellular messenger pathways and alterations in gene transcription and protein synthesis, alter the numbers and types of receptors and ion channels in target neurons, the functional activity of the intracellular messenger systems in those neurons, and even the shape and numbers of synapses the neurons form.

The figure is drawn to illustrate the amplification that intracellular messenger systems can give to neurotransmitter action. Thus, a single event of a neurotransmitter binding to its receptor (the first messenger level) can act through the second, third, and fourth messenger levels and so on to produce an increasingly wide array of physiological effects.

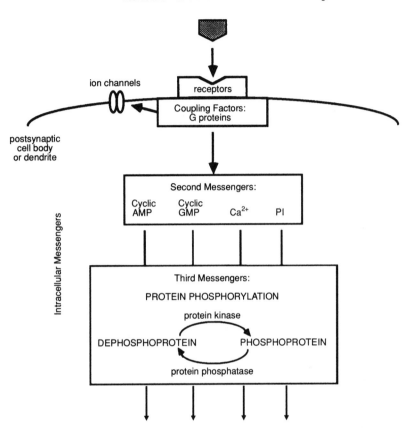

First Messengers:
neurotransmitters and other extracellular messengers

ion channels

receptors

Coupling Factors:
G proteins

postsynaptic
cell body
or dendrite

Intracellular Messengers

Second Messengers:

Cyclic
AMP

Cyclic
GMP

Ca^{2+}

PI

Third Messengers:

PROTEIN PHOSPHORYLATION

protein kinase

DEPHOSPHOPROTEIN   PHOSPHOPROTEIN

protein phosphatase

Multiple Physiological Responses

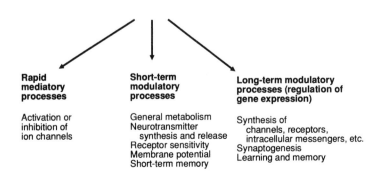

**Rapid
mediatory
processes**

Activation or
inhibition of
ion channels

**Short-term
modulatory
processes**

General metabolism
Neurotransmitter
  synthesis and release
Receptor sensitivity
Membrane potential
Short-term memory

**Long-term modulatory
processes (regulation of
gene expression)**

Synthesis of
  channels, receptors,
  intracellular messengers, etc.
Synaptogenesis
Learning and memory

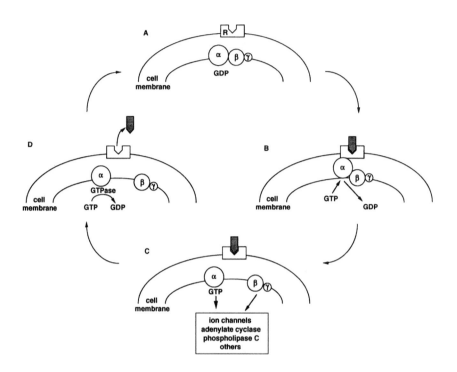

FIGURE 2–7.   Schematic illustration of G protein function in the brain. *A:* Under basal conditions, G proteins exist in cell membranes as heterotrimers composed of single α, β, and γ subunits and are not associated physically with neurotransmitter receptors (R). In this situation, the α subunits are bound to GDP.

B: On activation of the receptor by its ligand (e.g., neurotransmitter), the receptor physically associates with the α subunit, which leads to the binding of GTP to the α subunit and the displacement of GDP from the subunit.

C: GTP binding induces the generation of a free α subunit by causing the dissociation of the α subunit from its βγ subunits and the receptor. Free α subunits, bound to GTP, are functionally active and directly regulate a number of effector proteins, which, depending on the type of α subunit and cell involved, can include ion channels, adenylate cyclase, and phospholipase C. It is also possible that free βγ subunits directly regulate some effector proteins.

D: GTPase activity intrinsic to the α subunit degrades GTP to form GDP. This leads to the reassociation of the α and βγ subunits, which, along with the dissociation of ligand from the receptor, leads to restoration of the basal state.

sengers mediate the actions of neurotransmitter receptor activation on some types of ion channels (see Figure 2–5, C), as well as on numerous other physiological responses.

The molecular mechanism by which neurotransmitters regulate cyclic AMP levels is well established (Figure 2–8). G_s couples receptors (e.g., β-adrenergic; D_1 [dopaminergic]; and VIP receptors) to adenylate cyclase, the enzyme responsible for the synthesis of cyclic AMP, such that the enzyme is stimulated by receptor activation. In contrast, G_i couples receptors (for example, opiate, $α_2$-adrenergic, and D_2 receptors) to adenylate cyclase such that the enzyme is inhibited by receptor activation. The precise mechanism by which neurotransmitters regulate cyclic GMP levels is less clear, although it is possible that in some cases G_o mediates the ability of some neurotransmitters to activate guanylate cyclase (Figure 2–8). In other cases, nitric oxide appears to act as an intracellular messenger in mediating the ability of certain neurotransmitters to activate guanylate cyclase. The mechanism by which the neurotransmitters regulate nitric oxide synthetase and increase cellular nitric oxide levels remains unknown, but may involve Ca^{2+}.

Neurotransmitter receptor regulation of intracellular Ca^{2+} levels is more complex and can occur by two types of mechanisms that operate to different extents in different cell types (Figure 2–9). Neurotransmitter receptor activation can alter the flux of extracellular Ca^{2+} into neurons. This can occur in a number of ways: 1) Ca^{2+} can pass through ligand-gated channels, such as with the nicotinic cholinergic and N-methyl-D-aspartate (NMDA) glutamate receptors; 2) the conductance of specific Ca^{2+} channels can be altered by direct coupling of receptors to the channels via G proteins, such as with opiate receptors in certain cell types; 3) depolarization of a neuron by any means will activate voltage-dependent Ca^{2+} channels, which will lead to the flux of Ca^{2+} into the cells; or 4) activation of other second messenger systems can alter Ca^{2+} channel conductance; for example, cyclic AMP, and neurotransmitters that act through cyclic AMP, can increase the conductance of voltage-dependent Ca^{2+} channels.

Neurotransmitters can also increase intracellular levels of free Ca^{2+} through regulation of the phosphatidylinositol system, which can cause release of intracellular Ca^{2+} stores (Figure 2–9). Thus, many types of neurotransmitter receptors are coupled through G proteins to an enzyme termed *phospholipase C*. In some cases, subtypes of G_i and/or G_o are thought to mediate receptor activation of phospholipase C, whereas in other cases a novel subtype of G protein, termed G_q, has been implicated. Phospholipase C catalyzes the breakdown of phosphatidylinositol; this results in the generation of IP_3, which, through binding to a specific IP_3 receptor on intracellular organelles (e.g., endoplasmic reticulum), releases Ca^{2+} from intracellular stores.

The prostaglandin and leukotriene system represents an additional family of intracellular messengers that appear to play a major role in the regulation of signal transduction in the brain and elsewhere mainly by modulating the generation of second messengers. Prostaglandins and leukotrienes are generated as follows: The enzyme phospholipase A_2 cleaves membrane phospholipids to yield free arachidonic acid. The activity of phospholipase A_2 may be regulated by certain neurotransmitter-receptor interactions via G proteins, although this remains speculative. Next, arachidonic acid is cleaved by cyclooxygenase to yield, after numerous additional enzymatic steps, several types of prostaglandins and other cyclic endoperoxides (e.g., prostacyclins and thromboxanes) or by lipoxygenase to yield the leukotrienes. These endoperoxides and leukotrienes exhibit varied biological activity in influencing adenylate cyclase, guanylate cyclase, ion channels, and other cellular proteins.

Protein Phosphorylation as a Final Common Pathway in Regulation of Neuronal Function

Despite the large number of second messengers that can be activated within neurons, there is a relatively uniform way in which these signaling pathways

FIGURE 2–8 *(at right).* **Schematic illustration of the cyclic AMP and cyclic GMP second messenger systems in the brain.** Many effects of neurotransmitters and drugs, termed *first messengers,* on brain function are achieved through the cyclic AMP or cyclic GMP second messenger systems. Most neurotransmitters and drugs influence these second messenger systems through interactions with neurotransmitter receptors (R). However, some, particularly drugs (e.g., phosphodiesterase inhibitors, which inhibit the breakdown of cyclic AMP and cyclic GMP), can influence the second messenger systems directly. G proteins (G_s, G_i, or G_o) serve as coupling factors in that they mediate the ability of neurotransmitter receptors to activate or inhibit adenylate cyclase (AC) or guanylate cyclase (GC), the enzymes that catalyze the synthesis of cyclic AMP or cyclic GMP, respectively. These second messengers, in turn, activate specific types of protein kinases. The brain contains one major type of cyclic AMP–dependent protein kinase and of cyclic GMP–dependent protein kinase, although subtypes of these enzymes are differentially expressed throughout the brain. These enzymes phosphorylate a specific array of substrate proteins, termed *third messengers.* Cyclic AMP–dependent protein kinase has a broad substrate specificity; that is, it phosphorylates many substrate proteins and mediates most of the numerous second messenger actions of cyclic AMP in the nervous system. The substrate specificity of cyclic GMP–dependent protein kinase appears to be less broad, although by analogy with the cyclic AMP system, it is likely that it mediates many of the second messenger functions of cyclic GMP. Phosphorylation of the substrate proteins alters their physiological activity in such a way as to lead to the biological responses of the extracellular messengers either directly or indirectly through intervening fourth, fifth, sixth, etc., messengers.

NO = nitric oxide.

work. Although second messenger molecules may rarely have direct actions as effectors (e.g., cyclic AMP can bind to and directly gate ion channels in neurons in olfactory epithelium, and Ca^{2+} can bind to and directly regulate the activity of several enzymes), most of the known effects of intracellular second messengers are produced by stimulating the addition or removal of phosphate groups from specific amino acid residues in target proteins. Phosphate groups, by virtue of their size and charge, change the conformation of these substrate proteins, and in doing so change their function. For example, a phosphorylated ion channel may open more or less readily, a phosphorylated neurotransmitter receptor may be inactivated, and a phosphorylated neurotransmitter-synthesizing enzyme may act far more rapidly.

The regulation of protein function by phosphorylation plays a paramount role in signal transduction within the brain, a view originally proposed by Greengard and associates. In most cases, neurotransmitters regulate protein phosphorylation through second messenger–mediated activation of enzymes called *protein*

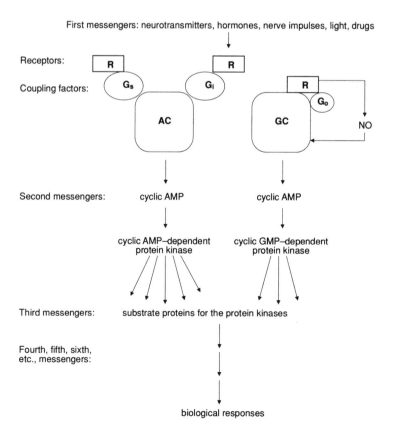

kinases. Protein kinases transfer phosphate groups from ATP to serine, threonine, or tyrosine residues in specific substrate proteins (Figures 2–8 and 2–9). In a smaller number of cases, neurotransmitters regulate protein phosphorylation through second messenger–mediated regulation of protein phosphatases, enzymes that remove phosphate groups from proteins through hydrolysis.

Protein Kinases and Protein Phosphatases

Among the most prominent protein kinases in the brain are those activated by the second messengers cyclic AMP, cyclic GMP, Ca^{2+}, and diacylglycerol. These protein kinases are named for the second messengers that activate them. The brain contains one major type of cyclic AMP–dependent protein

FIGURE 2–9 *(at right).*   Schematic illustration of the Ca^{2+} and phosphatidylinositol (PI) second messenger systems in the brain. Many of the effects of first messengers on brain function are achieved through the Ca^{2+} and phosphatidylinositol second messenger systems. As stated for the cyclic AMP and cyclic GMP systems in the legend to Figure 2–8, most actions of extracellular messengers on these second messenger systems are achieved through interactions with neurotransmitter receptors (R). However, some, particularly drugs (e.g., calcium channel blockers, lithium), can influence the second messenger systems directly. G proteins (G_i, G_o, and/or G_q) serve as coupling factors in that they mediate the ability of neurotransmitter receptors to regulate phospholipase C (PL-C), which metabolizes phosphatidylinositol into the second messengers inositol triphosphate (IP_3) and diacylglycerol (DAG). IP_3 then acts to increase intracellular levels of free Ca^{2+} (also a second messenger in the brain) by releasing Ca^{2+} from internal stores. Increased levels of intracellular Ca^{2+} also result from the flux of Ca^{2+} across the plasma membrane through Ca^{2+} and other ion channels, a flux stimulated by nerve impulses and certain neurotransmitters. As discussed in the text, G proteins mediate many of the actions of neurotransmitters on such channels.

These second messengers, in turn, activate specific types of Ca^{2+}-dependent protein kinases, of which the brain contains two major classes. One is activated by Ca^{2+} in conjunction with the Ca^{2+}-binding protein calmodulin and is referred to as Ca^{2+}/calmodulin–dependent protein kinase. The brain contains at least five distinct types of this enzyme—1–3: Ca^{2+}/calmodulin–dependent protein kinases I, II, and III; 4: phosphorylase kinase; and 5: myosin light-chain kinase. The other major class is activated by Ca^{2+} in conjunction with diacylglycerol and various phospholipids and is referred to as Ca^{2+}/diacylglycerol–dependent protein kinase or protein kinase C; there are at least seven closely related variants of this enzyme present in the brain. Protein kinase C and Ca^{2+}/calmodulin–dependent protein kinase II have broad substrate specificities (as indicated by the multiple *arrows* in the figure), and each probably mediates many of the numerous second messenger actions of Ca^{2+} in the nervous system.

The figure also illustrates that some of the second messenger actions of Ca^{2+} in the brain are mediated through proteins other than protein kinases. Phosphorylation of substrate proteins or third messengers, by these various Ca^{2+}-dependent protein kinases, alters their physiological activity in such a way as to lead to biological responses either directly or indirectly through intervening fourth, fifth, and sixth messengers, and so on.

First Messengers: neurotransmitters, hormones, nerve impulses, light, drugs

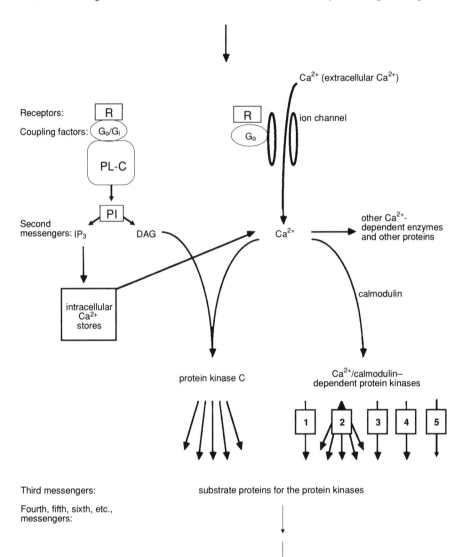

kinase and one type of cyclic GMP–dependent protein kinase (Figure 2–8), but two major classes of Ca^{2+}-dependent protein kinases (Figure 2–9). One is activated by Ca^{2+} in conjunction with the Ca^{2+}-binding protein calmodulin and is referred to as *Ca^{2+}/calmodulin–dependent protein kinase*. The other is activated by Ca^{2+} in conjunction with diacylglycerol and other lipids and is referred to as *Ca^{2+}/diacylglycerol–dependent protein kinase* or *protein kinase C*. The brain contains several subtypes of each of these Ca^{2+}-dependent enzymes, which exhibit different regulatory properties and which are expressed differentially in neuronal cell types throughout the nervous system. Cyclic AMP–dependent protein kinase, Ca^{2+}/calmodulin–dependent protein kinase II, and the various forms of protein kinase C appear to be multifunctional enzymes in that they each phosphorylate a large number of substrate proteins and thereby influence diverse neuronal processes.

In addition to second messenger–dependent protein kinases, the brain contains numerous other types of protein kinases. These include protein tyrosine kinases, which phosphorylate substrate proteins specifically on tyrosine residues, casein kinases, and a number of protein kinases that appear to be associated both physically and functionally with particular substrate proteins. It is conceivable that some of these also play a role in signal transduction in the brain. For example, protein tyrosine kinases are present in adult brain tissue at higher levels compared with most other tissues, show striking regional differences throughout the brain, are enriched in synaptic fractions of brain along with a number of prominent substrate proteins, and can be regulated by depolarizing stimuli and glucocorticoid hormones in discrete regions of the CNS. However, the precise role played by these various second messenger–independent protein kinases awaits more direct experimental demonstration.

Less is known about protein phosphatases than protein kinases, but it appears that the brain contains several types of protein phosphatases that differ in their regional distribution in the brain and in their regulatory properties. There are two known mechanisms by which neurotransmitters can influence protein phosphorylation through the regulation of protein phosphatases. One phosphatase, referred to as *calcineurin* or *protein phosphatase type 2B,* can be activated directly by binding Ca^{2+} plus calmodulin. Presumably, neurotransmitters that alter cellular Ca^{2+} levels influence the phosphorylation of cellular proteins through alterations in calcineurin activity. The other mechanism is indirect and involves a class of proteins referred to as *protein phosphatase inhibitors.* The best-known protein phosphatase inhibitors are phosphatase inhibitors 1 and 2 and DARPP-32 (dopamine- and cyclic AMP–regulated phosphoprotein, with a molecular weight of 32,000 daltons), the latter an inhibitor protein expressed predominantly in a subtype of neuron in the brain that receives dopaminergic innervation. These proteins are highly potent inhibitors of protein phosphatase type 1, and their phosphorylation by cyclic AMP–dependent protein kinase alters their inhibitory activity. Presumably, in neurons that contain these phosphatase inhibitors, neurotransmitters that alter cellular cyclic AMP levels influence the phosphorylation of cellular proteins through alterations in protein phosphatase type 1 activity.

Following the activation of protein kinases, or alterations in protein phosphatase activity, the next step in these signal transduction pathways involves regulation of the phosphorylation state of a specific array of substrate proteins for each protein kinase. These phosphoproteins are referred to as *third messengers*. A very large and increasing number of neuronal proteins have been shown to be regulated by phosphorylation. As shown in Table 2–5, brain phosphoproteins belong to every conceivable class of protein, indicating the widespread role of protein phosphorylation in the regulation of diverse aspects of neuronal function. This includes the regulation of ion channel conductance, neurotransmitter receptor sensitivity, neurotransmitter synthesis and release, axoplasmic transport, elaboration of dendritic and axonal processes, and development and maintenance of differentiated characteristics of neurons. As discussed in Chapter 4, phosphorylation of neuronal proteins plays a paramount role in the regulation of neural plasticity, including learning and memory.

The above discussion of signal transduction pathways portrays protein phosphorylation as the major molecular currency with which protein function is regulated in response to extracellular stimuli, a view supported by over a generation of research. Thus, although proteins are known to be covalently modified in many other ways, for example by adenosine diphosphate (ADP) ribosylation, acylation (acetylation, myristoylation), carboxymethylation, tyrosine sulfation, and glycosylation, none of these mechanisms is as widespread and readily subject to regulation by synaptic stimuli as phosphorylation.

Neurotransmitter Versus Neuromodulator

A distinction is sometimes made between a *neurotransmitter* versus a *neuromodulator.* According to this view, a neurotransmitter is a substance that acts through ligand-gated ion channels to directly depolarize or hyperpolarize the membrane, whereas a neuromodulator is a substance that acts through intracellular second messengers to produce more complicated effects. We disagree with this viewpoint and, in general, find the distinction between a neurotransmitter and neuromodulator to be arbitrary. First, as can be seen from Figure 2–5, neurotransmitter substances elicit postsynaptic potentials via three major mechanisms, not two. Thus, neurotransmitters can alter an ion channel by activating a receptor ionophore, by direct G protein coupling between receptor and ion channel, and by G protein coupling between the receptor, an intracellular second messenger, and ion channel.

Second, many neurotransmitter substances produce effects via all three mechanisms (see Table 2–4). For example, glutamate, GABA, serotonin, and acetylcholine each produce some of their postsynaptic potentials in target neurons via ligand-gated channels, but produce other postsynaptic potentials via G protein–linked receptors and intracellular messengers.

Third, it is not necessarily true that activation of ligand-gated channels has a more pronounced effect on the electrical properties of the postsynaptic neurons; there are examples in which a postsynaptic potential mediated via cyclic AMP– or Ca^{2+}-dependent protein phosphorylation has the most pronounced impact on target neuronal activity.

Fourth, as mentioned above, even though neurotransmitters acting through ligand-gated channels produce their initial postsynaptic potentials without the involvement of G proteins or intracellular messengers, activation of ligand-gated

---

TABLE 2–5.   Classes of neuronal proteins regulated by phosphorylation

Enzymes involved in neurotransmitter biosynthesis and degradation, e.g.,
Tyrosine hydroxylase
Tryptophan hydroxylase

Neurotransmitter receptors, e.g.,
Nicotinic acetylcholine receptor
β-Adrenergic receptor
α_2-Adrenergic receptor
$GABA_A$ receptor
Muscarinic cholinergic receptor

Ion channels, e.g.,
Voltage-dependent Na^+, K^+, and Ca^{2+} channels
Ligand-gated channels
Ca^{2+}-dependent K^+ channels

Enzymes and other proteins involved in the regulation of second messenger levels, e.g.,
G proteins
Phospholipases
Adenylate cyclase
Guanylate cyclase
Phosphodiesterase
IP_3 receptor

Protein kinases, e.g.,
Autophosphorylated protein kinases (whereby most protein kinases phosphorylate themselves)
protein kinases phosphorylated by other protein kinases (many examples)

Protein phosphatase inhibitors, e.g.,
DARPP-32
Inhibitors 1 and 2

Cytoskeletal proteins involved in neuronal growth, shape, and motility, e.g.,
Actin
Tubulin
Neurofilaments (and other intermediate filament proteins)
Myosin
Microtubule-associated proteins

Synaptic vesicle proteins involved in neurotransmitter release, e.g.,
Synapsins I and II
Clathrin
Synaptophysin

channels leads to multiple additional effects that are mediated via intracellular messenger pathways. Many of these effects may be as important, perhaps even more important, to the overall (particularly long-term) functioning of the brain.

Therefore, based on the original definition offered, a single substance can be both a neurotransmitter and a neuromodulator (and even something in-between), depending on the cell type, receptor subtype, and specific physiological response involved.

Heterogeneity in Brain Signal Transduction Pathways

As with receptors and ion channels, molecular biological studies have demonstrated extraordinary heterogeneity in intracellular messenger pathways, a degree of heterogeneity not suspected by classical biochemical, pharmacological, or physiological studies. For example, whereas biochemical and pharmacological studies indicated the existence of 4 types of G proteins (i.e., G_s, G_i, G_o, and G_t), 2 types of cyclic AMP–dependent protein kinase, and just 1 type of protein kinase C, molecular cloning studies now indicate the existence of at least 15 distinct G protein subunits, 6 distinct subunits of cyclic

---

TABLE 2–5.   Classes of neuronal proteins regulated by phosphorylation *(continued)*

Transcription factors, e.g.,	Histones and nonhistone nuclear
Cyclic AMP response element	proteins
binding (CREB) proteins	Ribosomal protein S6
Immediate early gene products	eIF (eukaryotic initiation factor)
(such as Fos, Jun, and Zif)	eEF (eukaryotic elongation factor)
Steroid and thyroid hormone	Other ribosomal proteins
receptors	**Miscellaneous, e.g.,**
Other proteins involved in DNA	Myelin basic protein
transcription or mRNA translation, e.g.,	Rhodopsin
RNA polymerase	Neural cell adhesion molecules
Topoisomerase	

Note.   This list is not intended to be comprehensive, but instead to indicate the types of neuronal proteins regulated by phosphorylation. Some of the proteins are specific to neurons. The others are present in many cell types in addition to neurons and are included because they have important functions in neuronal communication on development. Not included are the many phosphoproteins present in diverse tissues (including brain) that play a role in generalized cellular processes, such as intermediary metabolism, and that do not appear to play a role in neuron-specific phenomena. GABA = γ-aminobutyric acid. IP_3 = inositol triphosphate. DARPP-32 = dopamine- and cyclic AMP–regulated phosphoprotein (molecular weight 32,000 daltons).
Source.   Modified from Nestler EJ, Greengard P: "Protein Phosphorylation and the Regulation of Neuronal Function," in *Basic Neurochemistry,* 4th Edition. Edited by Siegel G, Agranoff B, Albers RW, et al. New York, Raven, 1989, p. 384. Used with permission.

AMP–dependent protein kinase, and 7 subtypes of protein kinase C. Such heterogeneity has been shown in each case to be due to a combination of the existence of numerous distinct genes for each of the proteins plus alternative splicing of some common genes (see Chapter 1). In general, comparison of the individual subtypes of these proteins has indicated that they possess different regulatory properties and exhibit varying levels of expression in different neuronal cell types. This high degree of heterogeneity indicates still greater potential for functional specificity within and between neuronal cell types in the brain. In addition, such heterogeneity raises the possibility of developing drugs that interfere with specific subtypes of intracellular messengers; these drugs would represent novel approaches in the treatment of neuropsychiatric disorders.

SELECTED REFERENCES

Berridge MJ, Irvine RF: Inositol phosphates and cell signaling. Nature 341:197–205, 1989

Bredt DS, Snyder SH: Nitric oxide, a novel neuronal messenger. Neuron 8:3–11, 1992

Cooper JR, Bloom FE, Roth RH: The Biochemical Basis of Neuropharmacology, 6th Edition. New York, Oxford University Press, 1991

Ferris CD, Snyder SH: Inositol phosphate receptors and calcium disposition in the brain. J Neurosci 12:1567–1574, 1992

Freissmuth M, Casey PJ, Gilman AG: G-proteins control diverse pathways of transmembrane signaling. FASEB J 3:2125–2131, 1989

Hubel DH: The brain. Sci Am 241:44–53, 1979

Hunter T, Cooper JA: Protein tyrosine kinases. Annu Rev Biochem 54:897–930, 1985

Kandel ER, Schwartz JH, Jessel T (eds): Principles of Neural Science, 3rd Edition. New York, Elsevier, 1991

Kikkawa U, Kishimoto A, Nishizuka Y: The protein kinase C family: heterogeneity and its implications. Annu Rev Biochem 58:31–44, 1989

Nestler EJ, Greengard P: Protein Phosphorylation in the Nervous System. New York, Wiley, 1984

Nestler EJ, Greengard P: Protein phosphorylation and the regulation of neuronal function, in Basic Neurochemistry, 4th Edition. Edited by Siegel G, Agranoff B, Albers RW, et al. New York, Raven, 1989, pp 373–398

Nicoll RA: The coupling of neurotransmitter receptors to ion channels in the brain. Science 241:545–551, 1988

Piomelli D, Greengard P: Lipoxygenase metabolites of arachidonic acid in neuronal transmembrane signalling. Trends Pharmacol Sci 11:367–373, 1990

Siegel GJ, Agranoff B, Alber RW, et al (eds): Basic Neurochemistry, 4th Edition. New York, Raven, 1989

Simon MI, Strathman MP, Gautam N: Diversity of G proteins in signal transduction. Science 252:802–808, 1991

Chapter 3

Overview of

Neuropsychopharmacology

Human interest in neuropsychopharmacology antedates modern scientific methods by centuries, perhaps millennia, as people in different parts of the world discovered that ingesting or smoking a variety of plant substances led to profound effects on their level of consciousness, sensorium, and mood. The ability to purify plant alkaloids with potent effects on the nervous system, such as morphine, cocaine, and reserpine, developed during the late 19th and early 20th centuries. The serendipitous discovery of the psychotropic effects of lithium in 1949 and the development of a large number of synthetic psychotropic compounds in the decades following have produced a powerful, although still imperfect, therapeutic armamentarium for the treatment of mental illness. Approximately 20% of all prescription drugs are given for the treatment of neuropsychiatric disorders. Similarly, a large percentage of over-the-counter medications, such as antihistamines and sympathomimetics, exert prominent effects on the central nervous system (CNS).

The concerns of neuropsychopharmacology are not only medicinal. It has been estimated that over 80% of the United States population uses some form of psychoactive drug for recreational purposes, mostly alcohol and tobacco, with 20% of the population abusing an illegal psychoactive substance at some point during their lifetime. Common drugs of abuse, in addition to alcohol and tobacco, include opiates, cocaine, amphetamines, barbiturates, marijuana, and hallucinogens. Between medical and nonmedical uses, psychoactive drugs have a major impact on the lives of many individuals and on society as a whole.

Text defined by vertical rules in the left margin involves advanced concepts and can be skipped by readers interested in a more general overview of the field, without loss of the overall message of the book.

UNIQUE FEATURES OF BRAIN PHARMACOLOGY

CNS pharmacology has important features that distinguish it from the pharmacology of other organ systems. One of the most important features is the blood-brain barrier. In most organs, substances dissolved in plasma can pass freely from the vascular space into the organ's extracellular fluid by diffusing between the endothelial cells that make up capillary walls. In contrast, the vascular endothelial cells in the brain form tight junctions with each other that exclude the passage of many substances into the extracellular fluid of the brain, that is, into the cerebrospinal fluid. An important feature of the blood-brain barrier is that foot processes from astrocytes make frequent contacts with the endothelial cells of brain capillaries. It is thought that some factor produced by these glial cells induces the formation of tight junctions by the capillaries during brain development.

A tightly regulated homeostatic milieu is absolutely necessary if the brain is to function. Without a blood-brain barrier, a small change in the concentration of ions in the blood, such as a fluctuation in serum K^+ or ionized Ca^{2+}, would markedly alter the driving forces on these ions into and out of neurons. A modest elevation of serum K^+, for example, would lead to depolarization of large populations of neurons and produce seizures. Similarly, because the major excitatory neurotransmitter in the brain—glutamate—is a dietary amino acid, ordinary meals might also produce prolonged seizures or neuronal cell death. The blood-brain barrier, which presumably arose through evolutionary forces, insulates the brain's environment from fluctuations in ions and metabolites as well as from most toxins. Relatively small changes in the brain's homeostatic milieu, which can occur despite the existence of the blood-brain barrier, have profound clinical consequences, as illustrated by states of delirium and toxic encephalopathy.

Ions and hydrophilic (relatively polar or charged) compounds are generally excluded by the blood-brain barrier. Such compounds can cross from the vascular space into the brain's extracellular fluid only via specific transporters that exist to transfer needed substances from the blood. To date, at least 10 different transporters have been discovered, including a transporter for glucose, the brain's preferred energy source, and 3 separate transporters for amino acids, one each for neutral (uncharged), basic, and acidic amino acids. Many of these transporters require considerable energy in the form of ATP. Indeed, the existence of the blood-brain barrier causes the brain to expend an enormous amount of energy in return for the careful control of the selective entry of a variety of molecules required for normal brain functioning.

In contrast to polar compounds, lipophilic (nonpolar or uncharged) compounds can readily cross the blood-brain barrier by dissolving in the membranes of endothelial cells, thus literally passing right through these cells. With the exception of lithium, essentially all compounds that are psychotropically active when given systemically are highly lipophilic. This requirement for lipophilicity has been a major obstacle to designing new drugs. Current research is focused on developing novel ways of delivering drugs across the blood-brain barrier. These include packaging them within lipid vesicles or attaching to them highly hydrophobic moieties that are cleaved from the drugs after they penetrate the brain.

Another distinguishing feature of brain pharmacology relates to the extraordinary complexity of the brain. As discussed in Chapter 2, the brain contains tens to hundreds of billions of neurons, each forming synaptic connections with perhaps thousands of other neurons. Each of the synaptic connections formed is not just "excitatory" or "inhibitory," but can exert complicated effects on its target neuron. Moreover, the neurons in the brain consist of thousands, perhaps tens of thousands, of distinct cell types with different functional properties. This is in striking contrast to most other organs, which contain at most a dozen or so distinct cell types. This degree of complexity makes the CNS very difficult to study. It also makes the treatment of neuropsychiatric disorders far more complicated, because a given disorder may involve primarily one or perhaps a few types of neurons in specific regions of the brain, thereby placing requirements for exquisite specificity on treatments for these disorders. The goal of an ideal treatment would be to selectively influence the affected neuronal cell type(s) without influencing any other neurons in the brain. In practice, such absolute specificity has not been achieved, which probably accounts for the high rate of side effects of presently available medications. One major focus of current research is to improve the specificity, and thereby the safety and efficacy, of psychotropic drug treatments.

Table 3–1 lists ways in which such specificity can theoretically be achieved. First, there are *anatomical differences* among neurons—for example, the loca-

---

TABLE 3–1.   Features that distinguish neuronal cell types and populations

Anatomical
    Location of cell bodies and projections
    Size, shape, staining properties
Pharmacological
    Type of neurotransmitter(s) used for synaptic transmission
    Types of receptors present on cell membranes
Molecular
    Numerous proteins or combinations of proteins
        distinct to different neuronal cell types that underlie unique
        characteristics of those neurons

---

tion of particular cells in the CNS. In theory, diseased neurons could be removed by surgery or replaced by transplantation. However, in contrast to degenerative diseases (e.g., Parkinson's disease), such approaches will probably not prove applicable to the vast majority of neuropsychiatric disorders, which may not involve anatomically well-circumscribed groups of neurons.

Second are what can be referred to as *pharmacological differences* among neurons. Neurons use different neurotransmitters for synaptic transmission and possess different types of receptors on their plasma membranes to receive incoming synaptic signals. Such differences in neurotransmitters and receptors represent the primary mechanism by which most currently available treatments of neuropsychiatric disorders exert somewhat selective effects on the nervous system. In the future, as molecular studies identify and characterize subtypes of receptors expressed in different neuronal cell types, it should be possible to develop drugs of ever-increasing specificity. A caution is that optimal treatment of certain disorders might require interactions with more than one receptor type. For example, the highly effective antipsychotic drug clozapine has less receptor specificity than typical antipsychotic drugs such as haloperidol. Whether this action at multiple receptor types is involved in the therapeutic mechanism of clozapine is unknown.

Third, there are *molecular differences* among neurons. What makes one neuronal cell type different from another must reside at least in part in different proteins expressed in those cells. For example, retinal ganglion neurons are different from cortical motor neurons, thalamic sensory neurons, etc., because each cell comprises a unique collection of proteins, some specific to that cell type, others shared by some other neuronal cell types. These distinguishing molecular features of neurons are only now being identified for the first time. They represent potentially novel means of influencing a particular neuronal cell type that might be involved in a mental disorder, for example, by selectively targeting a drug to that particular cell type. Finally, molecular biological studies also promise to identify the specific genetic abnormalities that contribute to major neuropsychiatric disorders in people, as discussed in Chapters 6 and 7. Identification of such abnormalities could lead eventually to measures, such as gene therapy, that can compensate for and even reverse the underlying pathophysiology of the diseases. Clearly, such a molecular neuropsychopharmacology lies many years in the future.

SITES OF ACTION OF PSYCHOTROPIC DRUGS

As mentioned in the Preface, studies of the actions of psychotropic drugs to date have focused largely on their effects on neurotransmitters and receptors. Most psychotropic drugs have been shown to regulate neurotransmitter synthesis, storage, release, reuptake, or degradation, or to serve as agonists or antagonists at specific neurotransmitter receptors throughout the nervous system. These various sites of action of psychotropic drugs are shown schematically in Figure 3–1. An understanding of the neurotransmitter and receptor systems in the brain has, therefore, formed the basis of the field of neuropharmacology over the past several decades and is the major focus of this chapter.

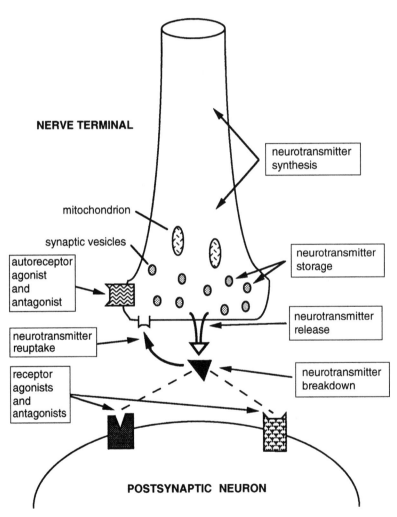

FIGURE 3–1. **Schematic illustration of sites of action of psychotropic drugs at the synapse.**

It is, however, important to note from the outset that this almost exclusively synaptic view of psychotropic drug action is inadequate for two major reasons. Most obviously, some drugs (e.g., lithium) do not exert their primary actions on neurotransmitters or receptors and have as their primary targets protein components of intracellular messenger pathways. (As pointed out in Chapter 2, the increasingly apparent heterogeneity of intracellular messenger proteins makes these proteins promising targets for development of future pharmacological agents.) More important, most of the actions of psychotropic drugs on neurotransmitters and receptors that have been identified by classical neuropsychopharmacological studies represent the immediate or acute effects of these drugs, whereas the clinical effects of most psychotherapeutic drugs are slow to develop and require chronic drug administration. For example, tricyclic antidepressants acutely inhibit monoamine neurotransmitter reuptake but do not produce their antidepressant effects for several weeks, and antipsychotic drugs acutely block dopamine (and sometimes other) receptors, but do not produce their antipsychotic effects for several days to several weeks. Thus, even when the initial interactions of a drug with its receptor(s) in the nervous system are known, the mechanisms responsible for its clinical efficacy usually remain unknown. It is likely that the delayed-onset therapeutic actions of drugs such as antidepressants, antipsychotics, and lithium are mediated by relatively long-term adaptations that develop in specific neurons in the brain in response to the acute effects of the drugs. Many of these adaptations are likely to be mediated by regulation of intracellular signaling pathways and neuronal gene expression. Understanding these long-term effects of psychotropic drugs on brain function lies at the heart of establishing a molecular approach to psychiatry and is the focus of Chapter 5.

PHARMACOLOGY OF MAJOR NEUROTRANSMITTER SYSTEMS IN THE BRAIN

As discussed in Chapter 2, a wide diversity of compounds serve roles as neurotransmitters in the brain (Tables 2–1 and 2–2). Throughout the CNS, the excitatory amino acid neurotransmitter glutamate and the inhibitory neurotransmitters γ-aminobutyric acid (GABA) and glycine are utilized at a majority of synapses. Via their receptors, most of which are ligand-gated channels (see Table 2–4), these amino acid neurotransmitters subserve almost all fast excitatory and inhibitory synaptic transmission in the CNS. This information has led to the view that projection systems using amino acid neurotransmitters represent the major circuitry of the brain that mediates rapid point-to-point information transfer. For example, afferent sensory information is rapidly conveyed from the periphery to the thalamus and from there to the cerebral cortex via glutamatergic pathways, and descending motor commands from the cortex to the motor neurons in the brain stem and spinal cord are also conveyed by glutamatergic neurons.

The other neurotransmitter systems in the brain consist of fewer neurons and, with few exceptions, involve G protein (so named because of their ability to bind guanine nucleotides)–linked receptors that mediate slower and generally longer-lasting changes in synaptic function. As a result, these other systems are often viewed as modulating the activity of the amino acid pathways in the brain. This is particularly the case for monoaminergic (noradrenergic, dopaminergic, and serotonergic) and many cholinergic neurons, which arise from a small number of cell bodies, localized in small nuclei in the brain stem or basal forebrain, and project widely throughout the brain and spinal cord. This anatomic organization underscores the view that these neurotransmitters represent intrinsic regulatory systems within the brain rather than systems involved in rapid point-to-point communication. This is consistent with the hypothesized role played by monoamines and acetylcholine in the control of level of arousal, attention, motivation, and mood.

Why has so much attention been focused on the monoamines and acetylcholine? Despite the fact that the monoamines and acetylcholine are utilized as neurotransmitters by only a low percentage of all brain neurons, they have been the focus of a high percentage of studies in psychopharmacology over the past three decades. Some of this focus is based on practical considerations: monoamines and acetylcholine were among the first neurotransmitters identified and remain among the easiest to study. From a more scientific point of view, this focus has some justification given the observations that many drugs that produce psychiatric symptoms or that are useful in psychiatric drug therapy interact with monoamines or acetylcholine, as will be seen later in this chapter. Moreover, based on their anatomy, monoaminergic and cholinergic neurons exert a pervasive influence on virtually all other central neurons, suggesting that they exert important modulatory effects on diverse aspects of brain function. Nevertheless, it is anticipated that a more complete understanding of the etiology and treatment of mental disorders will require attention to other neurotransmitter systems as well, particularly amino acid and neuropeptide neurotransmitters.

Inhibitory Amino Acids and the Benzodiazepine Receptor

Much of the original impetus to study the inhibitory neurotransmitter GABA came from attempts to understand the mechanism of action of the benzodiazepines, a class of widely prescribed drugs with anxiolytic, sedative, anticonvulsant, and muscle-relaxant properties. It is now known that GABA is the major inhibitory neurotransmitter in the brain, with perhaps 30% of all central synapses utilizing it as a neurotransmitter. It is not surprising, therefore, that the concentration of GABA in the brain is high: on the order of micromoles per gram of tissue, which is several orders of magnitude greater than most other neurotransmitters, such as the monoamines.

The chemical structure and synthetic pathway for GABA are shown in Figure 3–2. GABA is synthesized from glutamate specifically in GABAergic neurons by the enzyme glutamic acid decarboxylase (GAD). This enzyme has been purified to homogeneity and its gene has been cloned; multiple forms of the enzyme appear to exist in the brain. GABA is degraded by the enzyme GABA transaminase, which is localized to mitochondria. GABA is actively taken up by GABAergic nerve terminals, and this action, along with enzymatic degradation, appears to underlie inactivation of its synaptic actions. There are few psychopharmacological agents that interfere specifically with these aspects of GABA metabolism, although they are important targets for anticonvulsant drugs, many of which act by increasing GABAergic neurotransmission.

Anatomical studies in the brain using antibodies to GAD and more recent studies using antibodies to GABA itself indicate that the brain contains a multitude of neuronal cell types that utilize GABA as a neurotransmitter. These neurons range from small interneurons in specific layers of cerebral cortex to larger neurons of thalamus, caudate nucleus, and cerebellum with relatively long axonal projections.

The synaptic actions of GABA are mediated by two major receptor types, termed the $GABA_A$ and $GABA_B$ receptors. The $GABA_A$ receptor, the predominant receptor type, is the major receptor involved in fast inhibitory synaptic transmission in the brain. It is a ligand-gated ion channel: the neurotransmitter binding site is contained within the same multisubunit molecule as an effector ion chan-

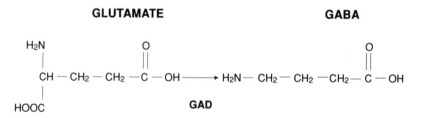

FIGURE 3–2. **Synthetic pathway for GABA.** Glutamic acid decarboxylase (GAD) converts glutamic acid to γ–aminobutyric acid (GABA).

nel (Figure 3–3). Because the channel within GABA$_A$ receptors is selective for Cl$^-$, activation of GABA$_A$ receptors hyperpolarizes neurons and thereby inhibits their firing. Given its inhibitory role in the brain, it is not surprising that the GABA$_A$ receptor is an important target of anxiolytic and sedative drugs. In particular it is the site of action of benzodiazepines, barbiturates, and some of the intoxicating effects of ethanol (discussed in Chapter 5).

The GABA$_A$ receptor is composed of multiple subunits, which have been denoted (based on cloning studies) α, β, γ, δ, and ϵ. The functions of the δ and ϵ subunits are not yet clear. The GABA$_A$ receptors that have been characterized are complexes of two α, two β, and one or more γ subunits. All of the subunits bear substantial sequence similarity to each other and to other ligand-gated channels (e.g., subunits of the nicotinic acetylcholine receptor and glycine receptor), suggesting that all of these receptors originated from a common ancestral gene by gene duplication and mutation. GABA$_A$ receptor subunits display an extraordinary degree of heterogeneity; to date, at least seven different α subunits, four different β subunits, and two different γ subunits have been cloned. The different subunits are differentially expressed in various regions within the CNS and display different functional properties. For example, in reconstitution studies in vitro, the different α subunits produce receptor subtypes with different affinities for GABA. In vitro, any pair of α subunits can associate with any pair of β subunits to produce a functional GABA$_A$ receptor, indicating that a very large number of receptor subtypes are conceivably possible. The actual combinations of different α and β subunits that occur in vivo are currently being studied.

The GABA$_A$ receptor exhibits a complicated pharmacology, in that it possesses several distinct binding sites that can influence the ability of GABA to activate its intrinsic ion channel. These binding sites, and some pharmacological agents that interact with these sites, are shown in Figure 3–3. The GABA binding site resides on the β subunit of the receptor; two molecules of GABA must be bound to open the Cl$^-$ channel. Muscimol is an agonist and bicuculline is an antagonist at this GABA binding site. It has been demonstrated by photoaffinity labeling that benzodiazepines bind to α subunits. *Photoaffinity labeling* means that the binding of certain benzodiazepines to the receptor becomes covalent on exposure to ultraviolet light; this greatly facilitated identification of the receptor α subunit as the benzodiazepine-binding domain of the receptor. However, the α subunit is unable to bind benzodiazepines unless a γ subunit is present; in other words, the γ subunit confers benzodiazepine binding on the α subunit, presumably by inducing a conformational change in the protein. Therefore, if GABA$_A$ receptors lacking a γ subunit exist in the brain, they would be insensitive to benzodiazepines. Benzodiazepines do not have a direct effect on

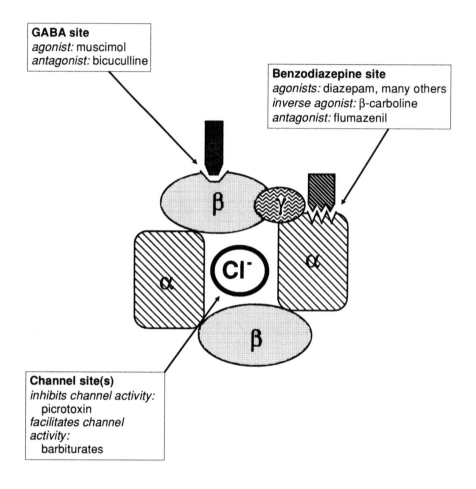

GABA site
agonist: muscimol
antagonist: bicuculline

Benzodiazepine site
agonists: diazepam, many others
inverse agonist: β-carboline
antagonist: flumazenil

Channel site(s)
inhibits channel activity:
  picrotoxin
*facilitates channel
activity:*
  barbiturates

FIGURE 3–3. **Schematic illustration of the subunit structure and pharmacology of the GABA_A receptor.** It is generally thought that all GABA_A receptors consist of two α and two β subunits, of which many subtypes are known to exist. In addition, some, and possibly all, GABA_A receptors contain one or more additional subunits, termed γ, δ, and ε (the latter two are not depicted in the figure). Three distinct binding sites have been identified on the GABA_A receptor. The GABA binding site, on the β subunit, is the site at which GABA binds and thereby activates the receptor's Cl⁻ channel. The benzodiazepine binding site, on the α subunit, is the site at which benzodiazepine agonists and inverse agonists bind and thereby facilitate and inhibit, respectively, the ability of GABA to activate the receptor. The presence of a γ subunit is required for the α subunit to exhibit active benzodiazepine binding sites. The channel site is located on the Cl⁻ channel domain of the receptor complex and may reside in the α and/or β subunits.

the GABA$_A$ receptor's intrinsic ion channel. Rather, benzodiazepines increase the sensitivity of the receptor for GABA (i.e., they increase the affinity of the GABA binding site on the β subunit for GABA) and thereby enhance the synaptic actions of GABA. This action is generally thought to mediate all of the clinical effects of benzodiazepines (see Chapter 5).

The GABA$_A$ receptor also possesses a binding site that resides at or near the Cl$^-$ channel itself. Picrotoxin binds to this site and thereby blocks Cl$^-$ flux through the channel and consequently the functional activity of the GABA$_A$ receptor. This action mediates picrotoxin's proconvulsant properties. Barbiturates and other sedative-hypnotics appear to bind to the same or some nearby site, but act to facilitate GABA-mediated activation of Cl$^-$ flux.

There is currently great interest in developing drugs with novel actions at the GABA$_A$ receptor. The demonstration of distinct GABA$_A$ receptor subtypes with different regional distributions in brain and different functional properties raises possibilities for the future development of drugs with improved clinical efficacy and greater specificity of action. For example, it might be possible to develop a nonsedating benzodiazepine for the treatment of anxiety, a sedating benzodiazepine to which no tolerance develops for the long-term treatment of insomnia, and an anticonvulsant benzodiazepine to which no tolerance develops for the long-term treatment of epilepsy. These possibilities are discussed further in Chapter 5.

Unlike the GABA$_A$ receptor, the GABA$_B$ receptor is G protein linked. It is not as widespread in the CNS as the GABA$_A$ receptor, but appears at least in some brain regions and spinal cord to contribute significantly to the synaptic actions of GABA. Activation of the GABA$_B$ receptor, through coupling with G$_i$ and/or G$_o$, has been shown to directly activate a specific type of K$^+$ channel and to inhibit adenylate cyclase activity. Because the driving force on K$^+$ is out of cells, activation of a K$^+$ channel would tend to hyperpolarize neurons, thus inhibiting their firing. Inhibition of adenylate cyclase would produce multiple actions on the target neuron. Baclofen, an agonist at the GABA$_B$ receptor, is used clinically as a muscle relaxant and in the treatment of spasticity; phaclofen is an antagonist at the GABA$_B$ receptor, but has no current clinical uses.

Much less is known about the glycine neurotransmitter system compared with GABA. Little information is available, for example, concerning the metabolism of glycine in its role as a neurotransmitter, as opposed to its function as an amino acid in general intermediary metabolism. Nevertheless, glycine appears to be a major inhibitory neurotransmitter, particularly in the mammalian brain stem and spinal cord.

The glycine receptor has been cloned. It consists of a pentamer of α and β subunits that form an intrinsic channel. Like the GABA$_A$ receptor, it is a ligand-gated channel selective for Cl⁻; activation of the channel hyperpolarizes and thereby inhibits neurons. Four different forms of the α subunit and one of the β subunit have been identified to date. Strychnine is an antagonist of glycine receptor function, an action that accounts for its proconvulsant properties. A second unrelated glycine receptor serves as a positive allosteric regulator of the NMDA glutamate receptor (see below).

Excitatory Amino Acids

A neurotransmitter role for glutamate was first established in invertebrates, where the compound mediates synaptic transmission at the neuromuscular junction. In more recent years, it has become apparent that glutamate also plays a major role in the mammalian brain. Indeed, glutamate is the major excitatory neurotransmitter throughout the mammalian CNS. The amino acid aspartate is also thought to function as an excitatory neurotransmitter, but its actions are still poorly characterized.

One of the major obstacles to the study of glutamate (and other excitatory amino acids) as neurotransmitters is the difficulty in distinguishing the relatively small fraction of glutamate involved in synaptic transmission from the much larger fraction involved in intermediary metabolism and protein synthesis. Although it is known, for example, that glutamate can be synthesized by several metabolic pathways, the relative contribution of each pathway to the synthesis of neurotransmitter glutamate is currently unknown. Similarly, the degradative pathways for glutamate, relevant to its synaptic function, remain unclear. Specific glutamate transporter proteins have been identified both in glutamate-containing synaptic vesicles and in nerve terminal membranes. Presumably, the former contribute to the ability of glutamatergic neurons to concentrate glutamate and prepare it for synaptic release, whereas the latter contribute to the inactivation of the glutamate synaptic signal.

Most important, the difficulty in identifying the specific neurotransmitter pool of glutamate has impeded progress in delineating the precise synaptic pathways in the brain subserved by this amino acid. Nevertheless, it appears that numerous and diverse neuronal cell types utilize glutamate as a neurotransmitter. Examples of well-studied glutamatergic cell types are granule cells in the cerebellum, pyramidal cells in the hippocampus, cortical motor neurons, and cortical neurons that project to the basal ganglia.

The classification of glutamate receptor types is in flux. In the most widely accepted current nomenclature based on pharmacology, the receptors are defined by selective agonists. One receptor type, the NMDA receptor (named for the agonist *N*-methyl-ᴅ-aspartate), has special properties (discussed below), including an intrinsic channel that can admit both Na^+ and Ca^{2+}. The remaining glutamate receptors are often lumped together as non-NMDA receptor types.

At least six non-NMDA glutamate receptor subunits and more recently several NMDA receptor subunits have been identified on the basis of molecular cloning. The relationship between these cloned subunits and pharmacologically defined receptor types (shown in Table 3–2) remains to be clarified. The pharmacologically defined non-NMDA receptors are the AMPA receptor (named for α-amino-3-hydroxy-5-methyl-4-isoxalone propionic acid; previously called the quisqualate receptor) and the kainate receptor. An additional receptor defined by the agonist L-amino-4-phosphonobutanoate (L-AP4) has also been proposed. These non-NMDA glutamate receptors are ligand-gated channels that are relatively selective for Na^+: their activation leads to Na^+ entry and subsequent membrane depolarization. They may also admit Ca^{2+} under certain circumstances. Non-NMDA glutamate receptors appear to be responsible for most of the fast excitatory neurotransmission in the mammalian CNS. In contrast to these ligand-gated channels, one type of glutamate receptor, of which two forms have recently been cloned, is linked by a G protein to second messenger systems (see Chapter 2). The functional role of these receptors, referred to as metabotropic glutamate receptors, is not yet well characterized.

NMDA receptors and excitotoxicity.   NMDA receptors have recently been a major focus of investigation because they have been implicated in a potential mechanism of memory called *long-term potentiation* (discussed in Chapter 5) and also because they may play a pivotal role in the death of nerve cells under condi-

TABLE 3–2.   Pharmacology of the glutamate system

	Receptor type			
	NMDA	**AMPA**	**Kainate**	**Metabotropic**
Agonists	NMDA	AMPA Quisqualate	Kainate	Quisqualate
Antagonists				
At glutamate binding site	AP5	CNQX	CNQX	AP3
At or near channel	PCP MK-801 Mg^{2+}			

Note.   NMDA = *N*-methyl-D-aspartate. AMPA = α-amino-3-hydroxy-5-methyl-4-isoxalone propionic acid. AP5 = D-2-amino-5-phosphonovalerate. CNQX = 6-cyano-7-nitroquinoxaline-2,3-dione. AP3 = 2-amino-3-phosphonopropionate. PCP = phencyclidine.

tions of anoxia or hypoglycemia. The NMDA receptor is a ligand-gated channel, but it has special properties not shared by other glutamate receptors. It has a number of distinct, pharmacologically important binding sites, and, as mentioned above, its ion channel is nonselective, allowing the entry of both Na^+ and Ca^{2+} (Figure 3–4). Recent cloning studies indicate that multiple subtypes of the NMDA receptor may exist in the brain, although more detailed characterization of the cloned proteins is needed.

The NMDA receptor has a binding site for glutamate, which can be antagonized competitively by d-2-amino-5-phosphonovalerate (AP5 [or APV]). The NMDA receptor also contains a binding site for glycine, which is unrelated to the inhibitory glycine receptor discussed above (e.g., it is not antagonized by strychnine). Glycine binding to the NMDA receptor alters the conformation of the receptor in such a way that glutamate can activate the ion channel. In fact, it appears that the channel cannot be activated in the absence of glycine. However, the binding of both glutamate and glycine is still not sufficient for the NMDA receptor channel to open. At resting membrane potential, the NMDA receptor ion channel is blocked by Mg^{2+} ions. Only when the membrane is depolarized (e.g., by the activation of AMPA or kainate receptors on the same postsynaptic neuron) is the Mg^{2+} block relieved. This arrangement gives the NMDA receptor very particular requirements for activation, which involve both the presynaptic and postsynaptic neurons. The presynaptic neuron must release glutamate to bind to the NMDA receptor, and the postsynaptic cell must be depolarized. Under these conditions, the NMDA receptor channel will open and admit both Na^+ and Ca^{2+}.

With anoxia or hypoglycemia, the highly energy dependent uptake mechanisms that keep glutamate compartmentalized in presynaptic terminals fail. Within minutes, glutamate is dumped into synapses, resulting in the activation of excitatory amino acid receptors. This leads to depolarization of target neurons via AMPA and kainate receptors and then to inappropriate and excessive activation of NMDA receptors. It is thought that large excesses of Ca^{2+} entering cells via the NMDA receptor channel are the proximate cause of the rapid cell death that occurs with anoxia. When present at high levels within neurons, Ca^{2+} activates a variety of enzymes, including proteases (enzymes that degrade proteins), and cells begin to "autodigest." Glutamate receptor–mediated killing of neurons has been termed *excitotoxicity.* In some animal models of anoxia or hypoglycemia and in neuronal cell cultures deprived of oxygen, neuronal cell death can be prevented by drugs that block the NMDA receptor channel. In other words, animals pretreated with such drugs, which are sometimes described as *neuroprotective agents,* may survive periods of anoxia with reduced brain damage.

The search for effective neuroprotective compounds that would protect the brain from glutamate excitotoxicity has converged serendipitously with psy-

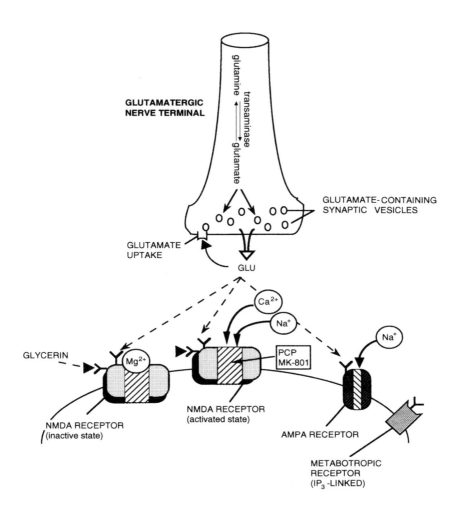

FIGURE 3–4.   Schematic illustration of excitatory amino acid receptors. The *N*-methyl-D-aspartate (NMDA) receptor on the *left* is drawn to illustrate blockade of the channel by Mg^{2+} ions. With depolarization of the postsynaptic membrane (for example, by activation of an α-amino-3-hydroxy-5-methyl-4-isoxalone propionic acid (AMPA) receptor channel, which admits Na^+ as shown on the *right*), the Mg^{2+} block is relieved as shown for the NMDA receptor in the *center*. If both glutamate (GLU) and glycine are bound at a time when the membrane is adequately depolarized, cations (both Na^+ and Ca^{2+}) can enter the channel. Phencyclidine (PCP) binds to a site located at or near the ion channel and blocks the functional activity of the NMDA receptor channel.

IP_3 = inositol triphosphate.

chopharmacology. In the search for nonaddictive opioid analgesics, a class of compounds called *benzomorphan opioids* was synthesized. These compounds, which include the approved analgesic pentazocine, produce analgesia by interacting with the κ opiate receptor (described below). However, certain benzomorphan compounds were found to produce psychotic symptoms even at low doses. Based on the actions of a prototype benzomorphan compound, SKF 10047, the psychotomimetic properties of these drugs are now known to be attributable to two independent binding sites, neither of which is considered to be an opiate receptor any longer. One of these sites is called the *sigma (σ)* receptor, but may actually represent some type of Ca^{2+} channel rather than an actual neurotransmitter receptor. The other site is identical to the site at which the abused drug phencyclidine (PCP) acts and is now often referred to as the *PCP receptor*. With additional analysis it was shown that the PCP receptor is a site within the NMDA receptor channel. Drugs such as PCP, ketamine, and the experimental drug dizocilpine (previously called MK-801), which bind at this site, are considered noncompetitive receptor antagonists and inhibit NMDA receptor channel function. Drugs of this type have been shown to protect neurons from death in a variety of experimental paradigms, including some conditions of anoxia and hypoglycemia. Unfortunately, these noncompetitive NMDA antagonists have serious behavioral consequences that limit their clinical utility. The search for nonpsychotomimetic, neuroprotective drugs has recently focused on other compounds that interact with the channel domain of the NMDA receptor and on antagonists of glycine at its modulatory site on the NMDA receptor.

The psychotomimetic actions of PCP have raised the question of a role for NMDA receptors in the pathogenesis of psychotic disorders. Very few relevant data are currently available, but it appears that glutamate and dopamine pathways have important interactions that may contribute to the etiology and/or pathophysiology of both movement and psychiatric disorders.

Catecholamines

The catecholamine neurotransmitters, which include dopamine, norepinephrine, and epinephrine, were among the first substances shown to act as neurotransmitters in the mammalian brain. Early research on catecholamines was greatly facilitated by the formaldehyde-fluorescence technique of Falck and Hillarp, which permitted direct visualization of both catecholamines and serotonin in the CNS. Catecholamines are synthesized from the amino acid tyrosine by a series of enzymatic reactions (Figure 3–5). Like most amino acids, tyrosine does not cross the blood-brain barrier passively and instead must be taken up into the brain by an active transport process. Catecholaminergic neurons contain the enzyme tyrosine hydroxylase, which catalyzes the conversion of tyrosine to dopa, the first step in the biosynthesis of the catecholamines. Dopa is then converted to dopamine by aromatic amino acid decarboxylase (often called dopa decarboxylase). In dopaminergic neurons, there are no additional enzymes in the pathway, and dopamine is the final product. In noradrenergic and adrenergic neurons, there is an additional enzyme, dopamine β-hydroxylase, which converts dopamine to norepinephrine. In adrenergic neurons, there is yet one additional enzyme, phenylethanolamine-*N*-methyltransferase (PNMT), which converts norepinephrine to epinephrine.

Tyrosine hydroxylase is the rate-limiting enzyme of catecholamine synthesis; that is, the other enzymes in the catecholamine pathway have higher activity than tyrosine hydroxylase and, as a result, do not limit the rate at which cate-

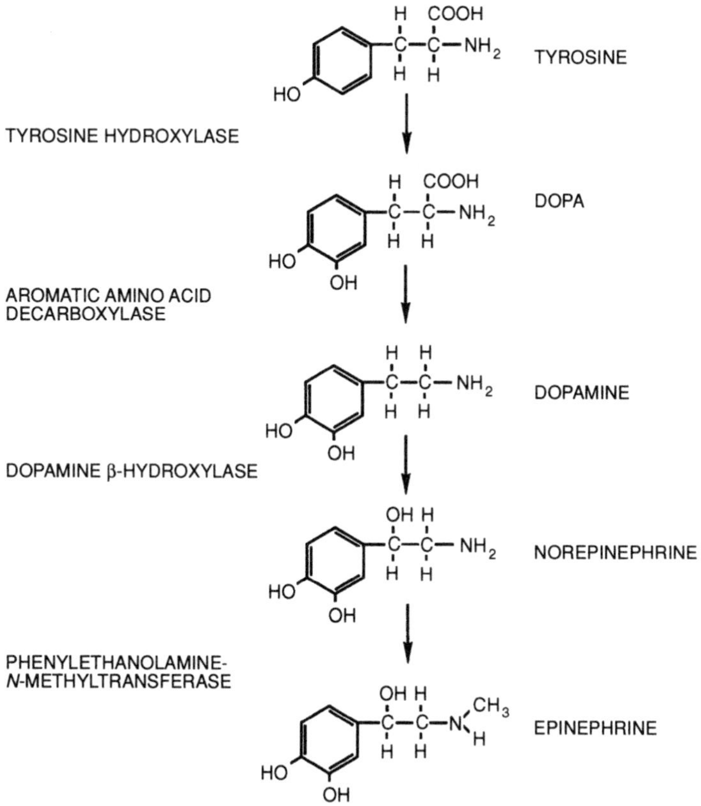

FIGURE 3–5. Synthetic pathway for catecholamines.

cholamines are synthesized. This means that the conversion of tyrosine to dopa by tyrosine hydroxylase is the critical control point in determining the rate of catecholamine biosynthesis. Because tyrosine hydroxylase exists at relatively low levels and, under normal conditions, is already supersaturated by the amount of tyrosine found in the brain, it is very difficult to influence brain catecholamine synthesis through variations in dietary tyrosine. Instead, the synthesis of catecholamines is largely controlled by processes that regulate both the activity and the total amount of tyrosine hydroxylase present in neurons.

In the short term, the activity of tyrosine hydroxylase is regulated by its phosphorylation by three distinct protein kinases—cyclic AMP–dependent protein kinase, Ca^{2+}/calmodulin–dependent protein kinase II, and protein kinase C. These kinases phosphorylate the enzyme on some shared and some distinct serine residues. In each case, such phosphorylation of the enzyme leads to its activation and appears to mediate the ability of neuronal activity and certain neurotransmitters, acting through the cyclic AMP and Ca^{2+} systems, to increase catecholamine biosynthesis in vivo. It is also likely that tyrosine hydroxylase activity is regulated in the nervous system through its phosphorylation by additional protein kinases. This is discussed further in Chapter 4.

In the long term, the total amount of tyrosine hydroxylase can be up- or down-regulated in response to a number of behavioral and pharmacological manipulations. Such long-term regulation of tyrosine hydroxylase represents

FIGURE 3–6 *(at right)*.   Hypothetical dopaminergic synapse. Dopamine (DA) is synthesized from tyrosine by the cascade of enzymes shown in Figure 3–5, is packaged in small synaptic vesicles, and is released when Ca^{2+} enters the presynaptic terminal in response to a nerve impulse. Dense-core vesicles are also shown. These generally contain neuropeptide cotransmitters; for example, many dopamine neurons synthesize and package the peptide cholecystokinin.

Reserpine blocks the uptake of dopamine into synaptic vesicles and causes already-filled vesicles to leak. Amphetamine causes release of dopamine into synapses without depolarizing the synaptic terminal. It is likely that amphetamine releases dopamine from a cytoplasmic pool that is not packaged in vesicles. The synaptic action of dopamine is terminated primarily by reuptake. Cocaine blocks dopamine reuptake by blocking the dopamine transporter. Intraneuronal dopamine is degraded by monoamine oxidase (MAO); this mitochondrial enzyme is inhibited by the monoamine oxidase inhibitors (MAOI). Dopamine may also be inactivated by catechol-O-methyltransferase (COMT) located in the synaptic cleft. Postsynaptic D_1 and D_2 receptors are shown. Both are G protein linked– receptors, as described in the text, and are antagonized to different relative extents by all currently available antipsychotic drugs. D_2 receptors are also shown on the dopaminergic nerve terminal; these are termed *autoreceptors* and serve a negative feedback role by decreasing the amount of dopamine released in response to a subsequent nerve impulse.

TH = tyrosine hydroxylase. DDC = dopa decarboxylase.

one of the best-studied examples of transsynaptic regulation of gene expression, which is discussed further in Chapter 4. The tyrosine hydroxylase gene has been cloned. Interestingly, whereas only one messenger RNA (mRNA) product is formed from the gene in rats, four mRNAs are formed (by alternative splicing) in humans. The possible functional and regulatory consequences of these four enzyme transcripts are currently being investigated.

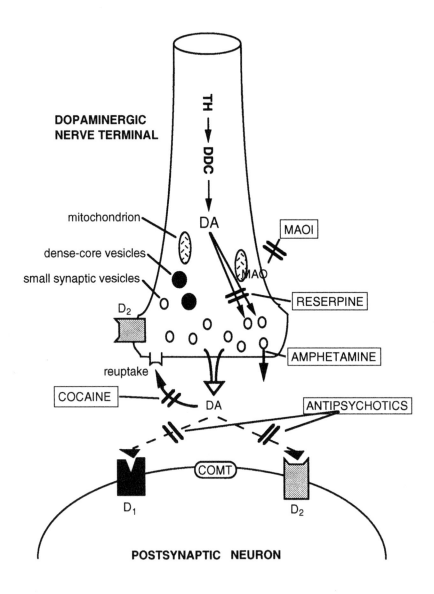

The primary mechanism by which synaptically released catecholamines are functionally inactivated is through an active reuptake process that transports the released catecholamines back into the nerve terminals. This is accomplished by specific transporter proteins present on the presynaptic terminal membrane. Once taken up, catecholamines are repackaged into neurotransmitter-containing vesicles for subsequent release. Catecholamines that are not packaged into vesicles are inactivated within the presynaptic terminal by the enzyme monoamine oxidase (MAO). There are two forms of MAO—MAO-A and MAO-B—both found associated with mitochondrial membranes within presynaptic terminals. Catecholamines can also be inactivated by the enzyme catechol-O-methyltransferase (COMT), which is located extracellularly. Schematic illustrations of dopaminergic and noradrenergic synapses are shown, respectively, in Figures 3–6 and 3–7.

As described above, the organization of monoamine (including catecholamine) neurotransmitters in the brain stands in marked contrast to that of the excitatory and inhibitory amino acids. Neurons that utilize monoamine neurotransmitters are organized into a small number of cell bodies that project more or less widely to cortical and subcortical targets in the brain and, in the case of norepinephrine and serotonin, to the spinal cord as well. It is important to stress, however, that although monoaminergic (and cholinergic) neurons project widely throughout the CNS, they do not release neurotransmitter diffusely into the extracellular space as has sometimes been taught, but appear to act, for the most part, at specific synapses. In addition, there is specificity of monoaminergic innervation of different regions of cerebral cortex and within cortical regions, even specificity of innervation of particular cortical layers.

Of the monoamine projection systems, dopamine has the least divergent set of projections (Table 3–3; Figure 3–8). Dopamine cell bodies are confined principally to the midbrain and diencephalon. The three major nuclei in the brain that contain dopaminergic neurons are the ventral tegmental area and the pars compacta of the substantia nigra, both located in the ventral midbrain, and the arcuate nucleus located in the hypothalamus. The nigral neurons project primarily to the neostriatum and form the nigrostriatal dopamine system. Antipsychotic drugs, which are dopamine receptor antagonists (see Table 3–5), are thought to produce their extrapyramidal side effects by antagonizing the actions of dopamine in this system. The ventral tegmental area neurons project primarily to limbic and cerebral cortical structures (e.g., prefrontal cortex, cingulate cortex, nucleus accumbens) and form the mesolimbocortical dopamine system. In rats, in which much research has been done, cortical dopamine projections are limited to frontal cortex. However, in primates, cortical dopamine projections are more widespread. Antipsychotic drugs are thought to produce their antipsychotic ef-

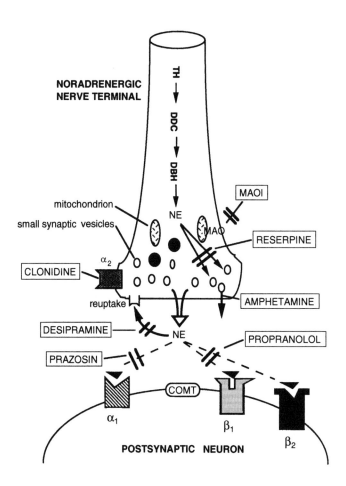

FIGURE 3–7. Hypothetical noradrenergic synapse. The synthesis of norepinephrine (NE) differs from that of dopamine by the presence of the enzyme dopamine β-hydroxylase (DBH). The effects of reserpine and amphetamine on norepinephrine storage and release, respectively, are the same as those for dopamine shown in Figure 3–6. Norepinephrine's action in the synapse is terminated by reuptake; this norepinephrine transporter is blocked by desipramine and some other tricyclic antidepressants. A variety of postsynaptic receptors are illustrated with clinically used antagonists. A presynaptic α_2 autoreceptor is also illustrated with the clinically used agonist clonidine. These noradrenergic autoreceptors serve a negative feedback role by decreasing the amount of norepinephrine released in response to a nerve impulse. All of the adrenergic receptors are G protein linked as described in the text.

TH = tyrosine hydroxylase. DDC = dopa decarboxylase. MAO = monoamine oxidase. MAOI = monoamine oxidase inhibitor. COMT = catechol-O-methyltransferase.

fects by antagonizing the actions of dopamine in this system. The arcuate neurons project to the pituitary and form the tuberoinfundibular dopamine system, which influences the release of a number of pituitary hormones. Antipsychotic drugs are thought to produce some of their neuroendocrine effects (e.g., hyperprolactinemia and galactorrhea) by antagonizing the actions of dopamine in this system. Dopamine is also utilized as a neurotransmitter by a small number of interneurons in the retina and olfactory bulb.

The major noradrenergic nucleus in the brain is the locus coeruleus, which is located on the floor of the fourth ventricle in the rostral pons (see Table 3–3; Figure 3–9). In contrast to dopaminergic neurons, which show relatively restricted axonal projections, noradrenergic neurons give rise to diffuse axonal

TABLE 3–3.   Localization of monoamines and acetylcholine in the brain

Transmitter	Cell bodies	Terminals
Norepinephrine	Locus coeruleus	Very widespread: cerebral cortex, thalamus, cerebellum, brain stem nuclei, spinal cord
	Lateral tegmental system and others in pons and medulla	Basal forebrain, thalamus, hypothalamus, brain stem, spinal cord
Epinephrine	Small, discrete nuclei in medulla	Thalamus, brain stem, spinal cord
Dopamine	Substantia nigra (pars compacta)	Striatum
	Ventral tegmental area	Limbic forebrain, cerebral cortex
	Arcuate nucleus	Pituitary
	Retina, olfactory bulb	Intrinsic
Serotonin	Raphe nuclei (median and dorsal) and others in pons and medulla	Very widespread: cerebral cortex, thalamus, cerebellum, brain stem nuclei, spinal cord
Acetylcholine	Basal forebrain: medial septal nucleus, diagonal band of Broca, nucleus basalis	Cerebral cortex, hippocampus, diencephalon
	Lateral tegmental area (dorsal pons)	
	Neostriatum	Intrinsic

projections and innervate virtually all areas of the brain and spinal cord. Mammalian brain also contains smaller collections of additional noradrenergic neurons and of adrenergic neurons that are located in discrete regions of the pons and medulla. These neurons show more restricted patterns of axonal projections.

Catecholamines exert their synaptic actions through a number of receptor subtypes, all of which show structural similarity to each other and belong to the family of G protein–linked receptors. The dopamine receptor types identified by classical pharmacology were termed the D_1 and D_2 receptors (Figure 3–6). Recently, D_2 receptors have been found to exist in two different forms, which differ only by a small number of amino acids. In addition, three novel dopamine receptors that were not predicted by classical pharmacological methods have been cloned. These have been termed D_3, D_4, and D_5 receptors. There is current excitement about the D_4 receptor because it has a relatively high affinity for the atypical antipsychotic drug clozapine, which is highly effective without causing extrapyramidal side effects (see Chapter 5).

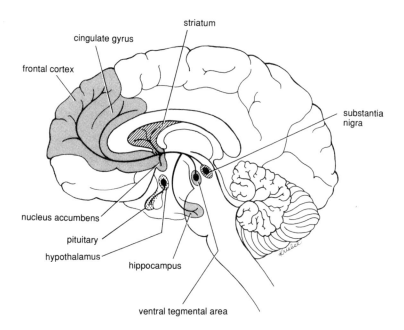

FIGURE 3–8. Dopaminergic projection systems in the brain.   The major dopaminergic nuclei in the brain are the substantia nigra pars compacta *(hatched)* shown projecting to the striatum (also *hatched*); the ventral tegmental area *(fine stipple)* shown projecting to the frontal and cingulate cortex, nucleus accumbens, and other limbic structures *(fine stipple);* and the arcuate nucleus of the hypothalamus *(coarse stipple),* which provides dopaminergic regulation to the pituitary.

In terms of primary amino acid sequence and pharmacology, the original D_1 receptor and the D_5 receptor appear to be closely related. Indeed, some groups prefer the nomenclature D_{1b} to D_5. Similarly, the D_2, D_3, and D_4 receptors appear to be closely related. It is possible that the dopamine receptor nomenclature will have to be revised to recognize these similarities. The D_1 and D_5 receptors appear to be coupled via G_s to the activation of adenylate cyclase, whereas the D_2 and possibly the D_3 and D_4 receptors are coupled via G_i and/or G_o to activation of a specific K^+ channel and/or to inhibition of adenylate cyclase, depending on the brain region involved.

Four main subtypes of adrenergic receptors have been identified—α_1, α_2, β_1, and β_2 (Figure 3–7)—each of which has been cloned. An additional receptor, termed β_3, has been cloned, but its function in vivo remains to be determined. In addition, there are indications that variant forms may exist for some of these subtypes with different regional distributions and functional properties.

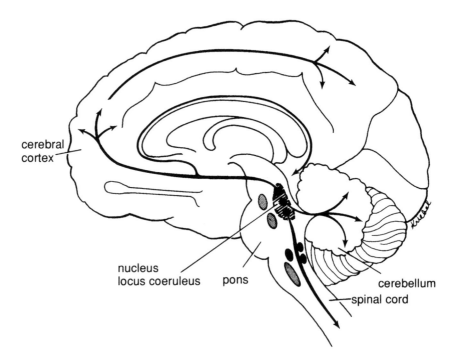

FIGURE 3–9. Noradrenergic projection systems in the brain. Shown are the major noradrenergic nuclei of the brain, the locus coeruleus *(hatched)* and the lateral tegmental nuclei *(fine stipple)*. Epinephrine-containing nuclei are shown in black. The projections from the locus coeruleus (as described in the text) are markedly simplified. Projections from the other nuclei are not shown.

Activation of β-adrenergic receptors leads to physiological responses by stimulating adenylate cyclase via coupling with G_s. Activation of α_1-adrenergic receptors leads to physiological responses through numerous mechanisms that, depending on the brain region, may include activation of phosphatidylinositol turnover. Activation of α_2-adrenergic receptors leads to physiological responses via coupling with G_i and/or G_o to activation of a specific K^+ channel and/or inhibition of adenylate cyclase.

A vast pharmacology exists for the catecholamine neurotransmitter systems. As shown in Table 3–4, drugs are available that interfere with the synthesis, storage, release, reuptake, and enzymatic degradation of these neurotransmitters. In addition, numerous agonists and antagonists specific for the various subtypes of catecholamine receptors are available (Table 3–5). These actions of the drugs underlie their usefulness in the treatment of hypertension (e.g., methyldopa, reserpine, clonidine) or Parkinson's disease (e.g., dopa, bromocriptine). It

TABLE 3–4. Pharmacology of the catecholamine systems

Site	Norepinephrine (epinephrine)	Dopamine
Synthesis	AMPT[a] (↓)	AMPT[a] (↓) Dopa (↑)
Storage	Reserpine (↓) Guanethidine (↓) Tetrabenazine (↓)	Reserpine (↓) Guanethidine (↓) Tetrabenazine (↓)
Release	Amphetamine (↑) Lithium (↓)	Amphetamine (↑)
Reuptake	Cocaine (↓) Nortriptyline[b] (↓)	Cocaine (↓) Nomifensine (↓) Mazindol[c] (↓)
Degradation	Pargyline[d] (↓) Tropolone[e] (↓)	Pargyline[d] (↓) Tropolone[e] (↓) Deprenyl[f] (↓)

Note. ↑ = drug increases process; ↓ = drug decreases process. AMPT = α-methyl-*p*-tyrosine.
[a]Methyldopa has similar effects on catecholamine synthesis.
[b]All secondary amine tricyclic antidepressants are relatively selective inhibitors of norepinephrine reuptake. In addition to nortriptyline, these include desipramine and protriptyline.
[c]Mazindol is a representative example of an increasing number of drugs that inhibit dopamine reuptake relatively selectively. However, mazindol appears to bind to a different site on the dopamine transport protein than cocaine, which may explain its weak psychostimulant activity.
[d]Pargyline is one of many available inhibitors of monoamine oxidase affecting both types A and B.
[e]Tropolone is an inhibitor of catechol-O-methyltransferase.
[f]Deprenyl is an example of an inhibitor of monoamine oxidase type B.

has also been proposed that such actions contribute to the mechanisms by which some of these drugs exert their clinical effects in the treatment of various neuropsychiatric disorders. However, as pointed out above, there remains considerable question as to how these acute actions relate to the clinical effects of the drugs that require their chronic administration. This is discussed further in Chapter 5.

Indoleamines

Indoleamines are synthesized from the amino acid tryptophan, which, like tyrosine, must be taken up into the brain by an active transport process. Serotonergic neurons express the enzyme tryptophan hydroxylase, which catalyzes the conversion of tryptophan to 5-hydroxytryptophan (Figure 3–10). 5-Hydroxytryptophan is then converted to serotonin by an amino acid decarboxylase,

TABLE 3–5. Pharmacology of monoamine and acetylcholine receptors

Receptor	Agonists	Antagonists
β-Adrenergic[a]	Isoproterenol[b]	Propranolol
α_1-Adrenergic	Phenylephrine	Prazosin[b]
α_2-Adrenergic	Clonidine	Yohimbine
Dopaminergic (nonselective)	Apomorphine	Most antipsychotics
D_1	SKF 38393	SCH 39166
D_2	LY 141865, bromocriptine	Raclopride
5-HT$_{1a}$	Gepirone, buspirone	
5-HT$_2$	Hallucinogens (e.g., LSD, mescaline)	Ritanserin[c] Ketanserin
5-HT$_3$		Odansetron
Muscarinic (nonselective)	Arecoline	Atropine[d]

[a]Selective β1 antagonists (e.g., metoprolol) are used clinically in the treatment of cardiovascular disease, whereas selective β2 agonists (e.g., terbutaline) are used clinically in the treatment of obstructive lung disease.

[b]These drugs do not penetrate the blood-brain barrier effectively.

[c]Some typical and atypical antipsychotic drugs (e.g., thioridazine, clozapine) have prominent antagonist activity at 5-HT2 receptors.

[d]Atropine is the prototypical muscarinic receptor antagonist, although others, for example, benztropine and trihexyphenidyl, are used clinically in the treatment of natural or drug-induced parkinsonism. In addition, a large number of drugs produce unwanted side effects by virtue of antagonist activity at this receptor: most tricyclic antidepressants and phenothiazine antipsychotics are mild to moderate muscarinic receptor antagonists.

which may be identical or closely related to the enzyme involved in the decarboxylation of dopa.

The rate-limiting enzyme for serotonin biosynthesis is tryptophan hydroxylase. However, this enzyme appears to be less limiting than tyrosine hydroxylase, indicating that, although difficult, it is possible to influence brain serotonin systems through dramatic variations in dietary tryptophan. Tryptophan hydroxylase and tyrosine hydroxylase appear to be subject to similar types of short- and long-term regulation. Such regulation presumably contributes to modulations in serotonin biosynthesis that occur in vivo.

Tryptophan hydroxylase is phosphorylated by Ca^{2+}/calmodulin–dependent protein kinase II and is activated on phosphorylation. In addition, there are indications that the total amount of the enzyme may be altered in response to chronic drug treatments and stress. One of the technical difficulties in studying the regulation of tryptophan hydroxylase has been the lack of availability of suitable antibodies. This difficulty should be addressed soon given the recent cloning of the gene for this enzyme.

As in the case of the catecholamines, the primary mechanism by which synaptically released serotonin is functionally inactivated is through an active reuptake process by which the released serotonin is transported back into the

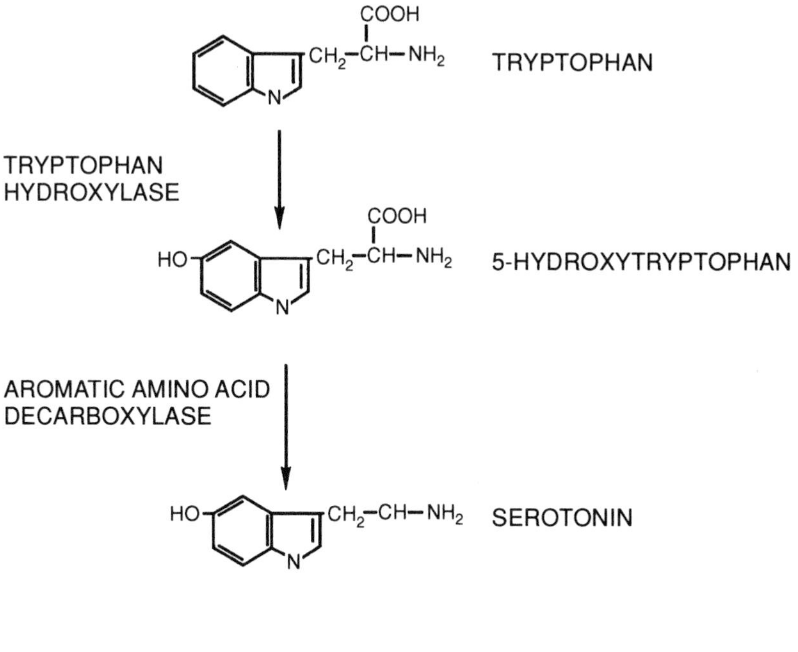

FIGURE 3–10. Synthetic pathway for serotonin.

nerve terminals by a specific transporter protein. Serotonin is then recycled for subsequent release. The reuptake transporters for dopamine, norepinephrine, and serotonin have received considerable attention because they are the primary, acute targets of a number of antidepressant drugs and cocaine (see Tables 3–4 and 3–6). These transporters, which have recently been cloned, represent distinct but related proteins. (All of the neurotransmitter transporter proteins cloned to date contain 12 membrane-spanning domains.) Like catecholamines, serotonin can also be inactivated enzymatically by MAO. As with the catecholamines, there are numerous pharmacological agents that influence the synthesis, storage, release, reuptake, and enzymatic degradation of serotonin. Examples of these are given in Table 3–6, and a schematic illustration of a serotonergic synapse is shown in Figure 3–11.

Neurons that utilize serotonin as a neurotransmitter are organized as diffusely projecting systems, with the cell bodies localized to discrete micronuclei in the brain stem raphe (Figure 3–12; Table 3–3). The two most important nuclei that

TABLE 3–6.   Pharmacology of the serotonin system

Site	Drug
Synthesis	PCPA ($\downarrow$) Tryptophan depletion[a] ($\downarrow$)
Storage	Reserpine ($\downarrow$)
Release	Lithium ($\uparrow$) MDMA[b] ($\uparrow$)
Reuptake	Imipramine[c] ($\downarrow$) Fluoxetine[d] ($\downarrow$)
Degradation	Pargyline[e] ($\downarrow$)

Note. $\uparrow$ = drug increases process; $\downarrow$ = drug decreases process. PCPA = *p*-chlorophenylalanine. MDMA = 3,4-methylenedioxymethamphetamine.

[a]A low-tryptophan diet, followed by a rapid ingestion of high levels of amino acids (other than tryptophan), has been shown recently to decrease brain levels of serotonin in animals and to induce a relapse in recovered depressed patients.

[b]MDMA, in addition to initially stimulating the release of serotonin from serotonergic nerve terminals, has been shown to be a selective serotonergic neurotoxin.

[c]All tertiary amine tricyclic antidepressants (e.g., imipramine, amitriptyline, doxepin) inhibit serotonin reuptake, but they are nonselective in animals and people because their secondary amine metabolites inhibit norepinephrine reuptake.

[d]Fluoxetine is an example of an increasing number of selective serotonin reuptake inhibitor antidepressants structurally unrelated to the tricyclic antidepressants. Others include paroxetine and sertraline.

[e]Pargyline is one of many available inhibitors of monoamine oxidase types A and B.

contain serotonergic neurons are the dorsal and median raphe. These neurons give rise to diffuse projections that innervate most regions of the CNS.

Serotonin exerts its synaptic actions through multiple types of receptors, identified originally on the basis of pharmacological studies but more recently studied by molecular cloning. These receptors, listed in Table 2–4, include G protein–linked receptors and ligand-gated ion channels. The different receptor types appear to produce their physiological actions through different intracellular messenger pathways. Some receptors, such as 5-HT_{1a} receptors in some brain regions, stimulate adenylate cyclase via G_s, whereas 5-HT_{1a} receptors in other brain regions are coupled via G_i and/or G_o to activation of a specific K^+ channel and/or to inhibition of adenylate cyclase. Other serotonin receptors, such as the 5-HT_2 or 5-HT_{1c} receptor, are coupled via G proteins to phospholipase C and the stimulation of phosphatidylinositol turnover; still others, such as the 5-HT_3 receptor, are ligand-gated ion channels. Examples of drugs that act as agonists or antagonists at these serotonin receptors are given in Table 3–5.

Uniquely in the pineal gland, serotonin is converted to the hormone melatonin via two enzymatic steps: one catalyzed by serotonin N-acetylase to form N-acetylserotonin, and the other catalyzed by 5-hydroxyindole-O-methyltransferase to form melatonin. In lower animal species, melatonin, released by the pineal gland according to a circadian rhythm, acts as a neurohormone to regulate skin pigment and reproductive function. The role of melatonin in humans remains unknown. It has been proposed to be involved in some forms of affective illness, although this remains controversial.

Acetylcholine

The pioneering studies by Loewi, Feldberg, and others established acetylcholine as the first chemical substance known to function as a neurotransmitter. Acetylcholine is synthesized by choline acetyltransferase by the acetylation of choline derived from phospholipids present in cell membranes (Figure 3–13). In contrast to the monoamines, the primary mechanism by which synaptically released acetylcholine is inactivated is through enzymatic degradation by acetylcholinesterase located in the synaptic cleft. Free choline is then actively taken up by a specific transporter protein in the cholinergic nerve terminals, where it is again acetylated to form acetylcholine.

In contrast to the catecholamines and serotonin, cholinergic neurons are organized in the brain both as widely projecting systems and as local circuit neurons (Figure 3–14; Table 3–3). The most important long-projection cholinergic neurons arise from nuclei in the basal forebrain. Neurons in the septal nucleus project to the hippocampus, and neurons from the nucleus basalis of Meynert and the diagonal band of Broca project to the cerebral cortex. Loss of cholinergic innervation of the hippocampus and cortex may contribute to difficulties with memory and to other cognitive deficits seen in Alzheimer's disease. In addition to a possible role in higher cognitive function, cholinergic neurons are thought to play a role in communicating the emotional state of the organism to the cerebral cortex. This inference has been made in part based on the observation that basal forebrain cholinergic neurons receive afferents from the limbic system and project to the cerebral cortex.

Other cholinergic neuronal systems are parts of local circuitry. For example, cholinergic neurons intrinsic to the neostriatum have important interactions with nigrostriatal dopamine neurons and striatal GABAergic neurons in the control of extrapyramidal movement. This cholinergic system is the target of anticholinergic drugs used in the treatment of both natural and drug-induced parkinsonism.

Acetylcholine exerts its synaptic actions through two major types of receptors: the nicotinic receptor and muscarinic receptor, named for the relatively selective actions of nicotine and muscarine, respectively, acting as agonists at these receptors. The nicotinic receptor, as discussed earlier, is a ligand-gated ion channel. It is composed of four distinct subunits, termed α, β, γ, and δ, and exists as a pentamer composed of two α subunits and one each of the β, γ, and δ subunits. Multiple forms of each subunit have been discovered. The receptor complex contains an acetylcholine-binding moiety and a nonselective cationic ion channel that is activated on acetylcholine binding. The nicotinic receptor is the

FIGURE 3–11 *(at right).*   **Hypothetical serotonergic synapse.** Serotonin (5-HT) is synthesized from tryptophan by the cascade of enzymes shown in Figure 3–10, is packaged in small synaptic vesicles, and is released when Ca^{2+} enters the presynaptic terminal in response to a nerve impulse. The effects of reserpine and amphetamine on serotonin storage and release, respectively, are the same as those for the catecholamines shown in Figures 3–6 and 3–7. The action of serotonin in the synapse is terminated by reuptake; this serotonin transporter is blocked nonselectively by the tricyclic antidepressants (which also inhibit the norepinephrine transporter) and selectively by the atypical antidepressant fluoxetine. $5-HT_{1a}$ receptors, which are G protein linked, are illustrated presynaptically as autoreceptors and postsynaptically on target neurons. The clinically available anxiolytic buspirone is a partial agonist at this receptor. The $5-HT_2$ receptor is also G protein linked as described in the text; ketanserin is a selective antagonist. The $5-HT_3$ receptor appears to be a ligand-gated channel. Odansetron is a $5-HT_3$ receptor antagonist, which is used clinically as an antiemetic. (The chemotrigger zone in the area postrema of the medulla is partially serotonergic.) Not shown in the figure are $5-HT_{1c}$ receptors, which share certain characteristics with $5-HT_2$ receptors.

TrH = tryptophan hydroxylase. AADC = aromatic amino acid decarboxylase. MAO = monoamine oxidase. MAOI = monoamine oxidase inhibitor. COMT = catechol-O-methyltransferase.

major mediator of cholinergic neurotransmission at the neuromuscular junction and in autonomic ganglia. In more recent years it has also been shown to contribute to acetylcholine's actions in some portions of the brain. Aside from nicotine, there are few drugs available that can cross the blood-brain barrier and influence central nicotinic receptors.

The muscarinic cholinergic receptor belongs to the family of G protein–linked receptors. It is the predominant type of receptor for acetylcholine in the brain. To date, four subtypes of muscarinic receptors have been cloned, designated M_1, M_2, M_3, and M_4, although it is anticipated that additional subtypes will be identified in the future. Muscarinic receptor subtypes show different distributions in the brain. In addition, they exhibit different functional properties in that,

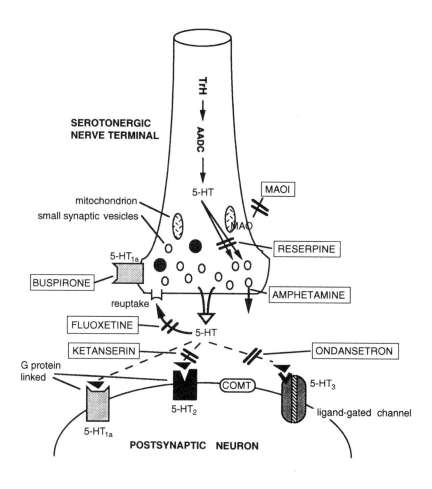

despite all being coupled to G_i and/or G_o, they exert differential effects on intracellular effector systems: activation of a specific K^+ channel, inhibition of adenylate cyclase, and stimulation of phosphatidylinositol turnover via activation of phospholipase C. Some pharmacological means of influencing muscarinic receptors are given in Table 3–5.

Cholinergic neurotransmission is a specific target of only a few drugs used in psychopharmacology, although the anticholinergic side effects of many drugs produce important problems in clinical practice (Table 3–5; Figure 3–15). In addition to producing familiar peripheral anticholinergic symptoms related to their effects on the parasympathetic nervous system, anticholinergic drugs impair short-term memory and in higher doses can cause delirium. Acetylcholinesterase inhibitors are used clinically to reverse the delirium caused by excessive doses of anticholinergic compounds. Physostigmine is the acetylcholinesterase inhibitor most often used for this purpose because it penetrates the blood-brain barrier effectively. Acetylcholinesterase inhibitors have also been used (thus far with very limited success) to improve memory in some cases of early Alzheimer's disease. Muscarinic receptor antagonists, such as scopolamine, are

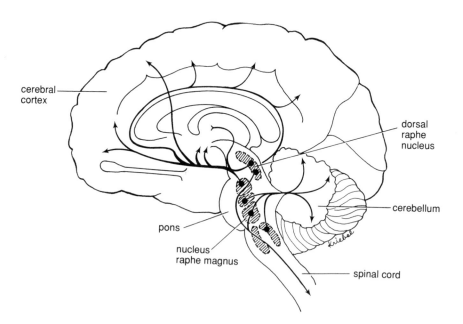

FIGURE 3–12. Serotonergic projection systems in the brain. The major serotonergic nuclei in the brain are the brain stem raphe nuclei (*hatched*). The nuclei are shown slightly enlarged and their diffuse projections (as described in the text) are markedly simplified.

used as over-the-counter sleeping pills and to prevent motion sickness. They are also used as antiparkinsonian agents, as mentioned above. The role of nicotinic receptors in brain function is not clear, but they appear to mediate the reinforcing actions of nicotine, the major addicting ingredient in tobacco smoke.

Neuropeptides

A large number of peptides have been identified in the brain. Most were already known from their functions outside the CNS, for example, as hypothalamic releasing factors (e.g., corticotropin-releasing factor [CRF]) or peripherally acting hormones (e.g., cholecystokinin) (see Table 2–2). Although some of these brain peptides have clearly been demonstrated to function as neurotransmitters, this has been difficult to establish with certainty in many other cases. To establish that a compound is a neurotransmitter, it must be shown that it is produced within neurons and released with depolarization of the presynaptic nerve terminal. Application of the compound to the postsynaptic neuron should mimic the results of presynaptic stimulation, and antagonists of the compound should block the effects of presynaptic stimulation. However, peptides are generally found in very low concentrations in the brain, which makes research particularly difficult, and very few antagonists of peptide action are known.

Anatomically, neuropeptides have an extremely irregular distribution in the brain: some peptides are found only in very restricted brain regions; others are distributed more widely. Peptides are utilized both by neurons that project for significant distances in the brain and also by local circuit neurons. There is currently some controversy concerning the distances in the brain that peptides can diffuse after release, because in many cases it appears that they are released

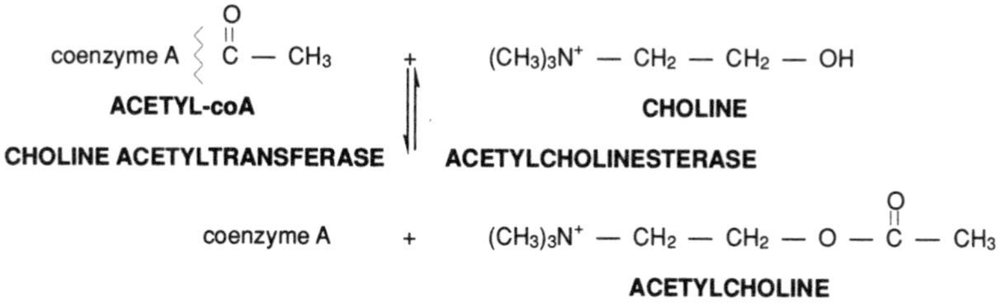

FIGURE 3–13. Synthetic and degradative pathways for acetylcholine. Acetylcholine is synthesized from acetyl coenzyme A (acetyl-coA) and choline. It is metabolized by the synaptic enzyme acetylcholinesterase. The chemical structure of acetylcholine is shown. (*Note:* The hydrolysis of acetylcholine by acetylcholinesterase produces acetate, not acetyl-coA.)

relatively far from neurons known to have their receptors. This has raised the possibility that peptides may function in some cases more like hormones, affecting a large number of target neurons over a wide distance, than like the classical model of a neurotransmitter, affecting one or a small number of target neurons across a defined synapse. A similar case has been made for the monoamine neurotransmitters, although the distances that neuropeptides and the monoamines actually diffuse in the brain after synaptic release remain to be established.

Unlike small-molecule neurotransmitters, which are synthesized by enzymatic pathways in both cell bodies and nerve terminals, neuropeptides can only be synthesized by transcription and translation in cell bodies. As will be discussed in Chapter 4, the initiation of transcription appears to be a critical control point in neuropeptide biosynthesis. It has been found that the nuclear mRNA derived from genes encoding certain neuropeptides can be processed in alternate ways in different cell types. By including or excluding particular exons in the mature cytoplasmic mRNA, mRNAs encoding distinctly different peptides can be produced. For example, calcitonin and calcitonin gene–related peptide are the products of the same gene derived by such alternate splicing. In some

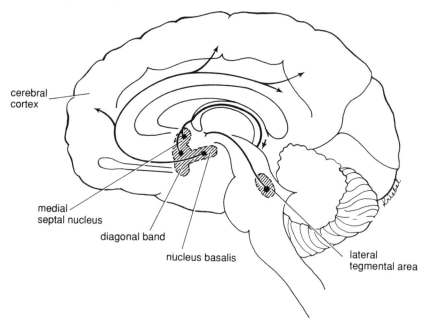

FIGURE 3–14. Cholinergic projection systems in the brain. The major, widely projecting cholinergic nuclei in the brain are shown, including a large group in the basal forebrain and a smaller nucleus in the lateral tegmental area of the brain stem. The projections of these neurons are shown markedly simplified. Local circuit cholinergic neurons (e.g., within the striatum) are omitted for simplicity.

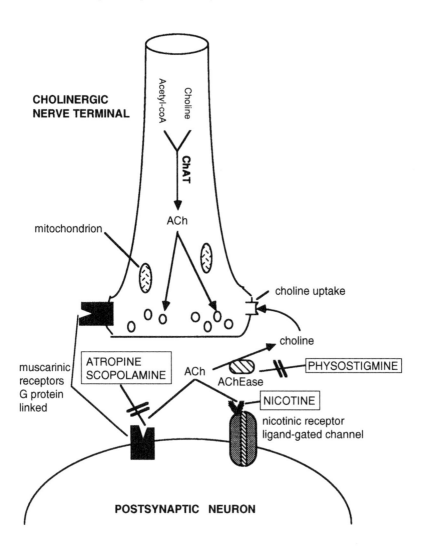

FIGURE 3–15.　Hypothetical cholinergic synapse. Acetylcholine (ACh) is synthesized from choline and acetyl coenzyme A (acetyl-coA) by the enzyme choline acetyltransferase (ChAT). In contrast to monoamines, which are inactivated primarily by reuptake, synaptic acetylcholine is inactivated enzymatically by acetylcholinesterase (AChEase). Physostigmine, an acetylcholinesterase inhibitor, increases the synaptic life of acetylcholine. There are two classes of receptors for acetylcholine: 1) nicotinic, which are ligand-gated channels, and 2) muscarinic, which are G protein linked. Within both of these classes there are multiple subtypes. Drugs with psychotropic effects mediated by cholinergic receptors are shown: two nonselective antagonists of muscarinic receptors, atropine and scopolamine, and the classical agonist at nicotinic receptors, nicotine.

cells in which the gene is expressed (e.g., medullary cells of the thyroid), the nuclear mRNA is processed to yield a mature cytoplasmic mRNA encoding calcitonin, whereas in neurons the predominant transcript encodes calcitonin gene–related peptide. Alternate splicing also appears to be an important mechanism of control for the preprotachykinin gene, which encodes both substance P and substance K. The degree to which alternate splicing is utilized for other peptide gene products is currently an area of active research. This mechanism, described in greater detail in Chapter 1, increases the diversity of signaling molecules that can be generated from a single gene. However, a particular pattern of splicing appears to be a stable characteristic of a cell type and not subject to regulation over time. It would appear, therefore, that different cell types contain distinct "spliceases"—ribonucleotide-containing enzymes responsible for mRNA splicing—although this possibility requires further study.

The mature mRNAs that encode neuropeptides are translated to give rise to large precursors. These precursors (e.g., preproenkephalin or preprotachykinin) contain a sequence, almost always at the amino terminus of the protein (the end that is translated first), that acts to target the protein to the neuron's secretory pathway. This leader sequence or "pre" sequence is rapidly cleaved by protease enzymes (sometimes termed "endopeptidases"), leaving the remainder of the precursor (e.g., proenkephalin or protachykinin). This precursor then undergoes further proteolytic cleavage and subsequent chemical modification (e.g., glycosylation, amidation, acetylation, or phosphorylation) to yield numerous biologically active peptides for release. Just as alternate splicing of mRNAs permits the generation of multiple signaling molecules from a single gene, differential processing of peptide precursors permits the generation of a wide diversity of signaling molecules from a single peptide precursor. Interestingly, the large precursors are often processed differently in particular neuronal types to yield peptides that may have strikingly different physiological roles. Such differences in processing may result in part from different proteases expressed in various types of neurons. Within neuropeptide precursors, the internal "signal" for proteolytic processing is pairs of basic amino acids, that is, some combination of lysine and arginine. Not all possible dibasic pairs are cleaved equally well by the different proteases found in cells.

Little is known in general about neuropeptide receptors in the brain, although an increasing number have been cloned. Certain neuropeptides, such as vasoactive intestinal polypeptide and CRF, appear to exert many of their effects through activation of adenylate cyclase via G_s coupling. Other neuropeptides, such as the opiates (see below) and neuropeptide Y, are coupled via G_i and/or G_o to numerous intracellular effectors. Still others, such as substance P, appear to produce their physiological actions via the phosphatidylinositol system.

There is currently intense interest in developing drugs that influence specific neuropeptide systems in the brain. One of the challenges is to synthesize molecules that are agonists or antagonists at neuropeptide receptors but that can pass freely across the blood-brain barrier. Such drugs would represent novel treatments for neuropsychiatric disorders. For example, CRF has been implicated in mediating some of the effects of stress on brain function. CRF antagonists could, theoretically, be of benefit in the treatment of affective and anxiety disorders. Similarly, cholecystokinin and neurotensin are colocalized with dopamine neurons in the brain, raising the possibility that ligands for these peptide receptors could be useful in the treatment of psychosis.

Opioid peptides.   Among the peptide neurotransmitters, the endogenous opioid peptides are the best studied. They are of importance to psychiatry because they function to suppress pain as "endogenous analgesics," may be involved in modulation of mood states, are very likely to be involved in brain reward and drug addiction, and appear to be involved in regulation of pituitary hormone release, as well as in many other functions.

Receptors for opioids were discovered by Goldstein, Snyder, and others in the brain as part of an effort to find the sites at which natural opiate alkaloids, such as morphine, act in the CNS. The presence of such receptors in the brain led to an intense search for endogenous opioid neurotransmitters, which were viewed as potential endogenous analgesic systems. Hughes and Kosterlitz first identified endogenous opioids in the 1970s, and over the past 15 years, at least 18 opioid peptides have been isolated and characterized from mammalian brain, pituitary, and adrenal gland by numerous laboratories. All of these endogenous opioids contain the same four amino acids at their amino terminus, Tyr-Gly-Gly-Phe, followed by either Met or Leu. Opiate alkaloids derived from the opium poppy appear to mimic the structure of the amino-terminal tyrosine in these peptides such that they interact with the same receptors. It has been found that all of the endogenous opioid peptides are the products of three large precursors, each encoded by a separate gene. The precursors are pro-opiomelanocortin (which is the precursor of β-endorphin, of adrenocorticotropic hormone [ACTH], and of α-melanocyte–stimulating hormone), proenkephalin (which encodes six copies of the Met-enkephalin sequence and one of the Leu-enkephalin sequence), and prodynorphin (which is the precursor of dynorphin and related peptides).

Endogenous opioid peptides and exogenous opiate alkaloids exert their actions in the nervous system via activation of specific opiate receptors. Three major types of opiate receptors have been discovered: μ, δ, and κ. Morphine-like opiates preferentially bind to the μ opiate receptor, whereas the benzomorphan opioids preferentially bind to the κ receptor. Of the endogenous opioid peptides, β-endorphin has the greatest affinity for μ receptors, enkephalins for δ receptors, and dynorphin for κ receptors. However, despite these rank orders of affinity, there do not appear to be separate endogenous opioid systems matching certain peptides with receptor types, because the differences in affinity are not so great as to be exclusive. Thus, in vivo, the determinants of which peptide stimulates which receptor depend not only on affinity, but also on the proximity of the various peptides to the receptors. Naloxone and naltrexone are antagonists at all three receptor types with the following relative affinities: μ > δ > κ.

Each of the three classes of opiate receptors show widespread distribution in the brain and spinal cord, and it has been difficult to assign a particular physiological role to a particular receptor. However, the μ receptor appears to be the most important opiate receptor involved in supraspinal analgesia, whereas the δ and κ receptors appear to be more involved in analgesia at the level of the dorsal horn of the spinal cord. To further complicate matters, pharmacological studies suggest that there may be numerous subtypes of each opiate receptor, with numerous agonists and antagonists showing characteristic affinities for these various subtypes. However, to date, no opiate receptor has been cloned or definitively purified, and this has greatly hindered efforts to characterize the diverse types of opiate receptors in the CNS and to study their role in mediating the actions of exogenous and endogenous opioids.

There has been great interest over the years in identifying the intracellular signal transduction pathways through which the opiate receptors exert their physiological actions. Indirect evidence suggests that all major types of opiate receptors belong to the family of G protein–linked receptors, although this awaits direct confirmation from cloning studies. It now appears that μ, δ, and κ receptors each couple with G_i and/or G_o to activate directly (depending on the cell type) a specific type of K^+ channel, inhibit voltage-dependent Ca^{2+} channels, and/or inhibit adenylate cyclase, which would then lead to numerous other effects of opiates in the target neurons. The acute mechanisms of action of opiates, and possible mechanisms underlying the development of opiate addiction, are discussed further in Chapter 5.

In addition to effects mediated by currently recognized opiate receptor types, certain opioid drugs, especially benzomorphan compounds (such as pentazocine), produce unwanted nonopiate receptor effects, including psychosis. These effects have been attributed, as described above, to two binding sites in brain, the σ and PCP receptors, neither of which is currently considered to be an opiate receptor because drug effects at these sites are not antagonized by naloxone. Clinical interest in the PCP receptor is discussed in the context of the NMDA receptor earlier in this chapter. Clinical interest in the σ receptor (likely some type of Ca^{2+} channel) has been heightened by the observation that certain, but not all, antipsychotic drugs (e.g., haloperidol) are potent σ receptor antagonists; that is, they block the binding of psychotomimetic opiates at these sites. A variety of drugs that are σ receptor antagonists, but not dopamine antagonists, are being tested for antipsychotic activity. If effective, such compounds would be antipsychotic with presumably little risk of extrapyramidal side effects that are due to dopamine receptor blockade.

SELECTED REFERENCES

Burt DR, Kamatchi GL: GABA$_A$ receptor subtypes: from pharmacology to molecular biology. FASEB J 5:2916–2923, 1991

Cooper JR, Bloom FE, Roth RH: The Biochemical Basis of Neuropharmacology, 6th Edition. Oxford University Press, New York, 1991

Foote SL, Morrison JH: Extrathalamic modulation of cortical function. Annu Rev Neurosci 10:67–95, 1987

Gasic GP, Heinemann S: Receptors coupled to ionic channels: the glutamate receptor family. Current Opinion in Neurobiology 1:20–26, 1991

Goodman RH: Regulation of neuropeptide gene expression. Annu Rev Neurosci 13:111–128, 1990

Julius D: Molecular biology of serotonin receptors. Annu Rev Neurosci 14:335–360, 1991

Levitan ES, Schofield PR, Burt DR, et al: Structural and functional basis for GABA$_A$ receptor heterogeneity. Nature 335:76–79, 1988

Moriyoshi K, Masu M, Ishii T, et al: Molecular cloning and characterization of the rat NMDA receptor. Nature 354:31–37, 1991

Nakanishi N, Shneider NA, Axel R: A family of glutamate receptor genes: evidence for the formation of heteromultimeric receptors with distinct channel properties. Neuron 5:569–581, 1990

Pasternak GW: Multiple morphine and enkephalin receptors and the relief of pain. JAMA 259:1362–1367, 1988

Pritchett DB, Sontheimer H, Shivers BD, et al: Importance of a novel GABA$_A$ receptor subunit for benzodiazepine pharmacology. Nature 13(338):582–585, 1989

Robinson MB, Coyle JT: Glutamate and related acidic neurotransmitters: from basic science to clinical practice. FASEB J 1:446–455, 1987

Chapter 4

Mechanisms of

Neural Plasticity

The human brain is remarkably plastic. It adapts to a wide variety of circumstances, forms memories of experiences, and learns procedures; it can become dependent on drugs or produce disabling psychopathology; and it can recover. The plasticity of our brains, and therefore our ability to learn and adapt, is at the heart of our evolutionary success in nature and of our cultural evolution as well. What are the processes underlying this plasticity?

Until relatively recently, synaptic transmission was narrowly conceptualized as a set of processes by which neurotransmitters, acting through their receptors, caused changes in the conductances of specific ion channels to produce excitatory or inhibitory postsynaptic potentials (see Figure 2–3). According to this view, the human brain could be conceptualized as a very complex digital computer with its complexity derived largely from its wiring diagram. Over the past 10 years, however, it has become evident that neurotransmitters elicit diverse and complicated effects in target neurons, which has led to a much more complete view of synaptic transmission (Figure 2–6). We now know that neurotransmitters may produce prolonged changes in the way that their target neurons process subsequent synaptic information. Unlike direct excitation or inhibition of postsynaptic neurons, such "modulatory" effects may not be detected until the neuron is stimulated again by the same or other neurotransmitters.

Two general types of biochemical mechanisms appear to underlie the modulatory effects of neurotransmitters. One is protein phosphorylation, whereby modulation of neuronal function is achieved through phosphorylation-induced alterations in the functional state of diverse types of neuronal proteins such as

---

Text defined by vertical rules in the left margin involves advanced concepts and can be skipped by readers interested in a more general overview of the field, without loss of the overall message of the book.

ion channels (which would alter the electrical excitability of target neurons), neurotransmitter receptors (which would alter the responsiveness of target neurons to synaptic inputs), and neurotransmitter synthetic enzymes and proteins that control neurotransmitter storage and release (which would alter the ability of the neurons to influence their targets).

A second general mechanism by which neurotransmitters can elicit long-term changes in the function of target neurons is by regulating gene expression within those neurons. Changes in gene expression may produce quantitative and even qualitative changes in the protein components of neurons. Some examples include alterations in the numbers and types of ion channels and receptors present on the cell membrane, levels of proteins involved in postreceptor signal transduction, and proteins that regulate the morphology of neurons and the numbers of synaptic connections they form. Regulation of neuronal gene expression by neurotransmitters occurs on a continual basis to fine-tune the functional state of neurons in response to complex synaptic inputs.

Ultimately, long-term effects of environmental factors on the brain, including long-term behavioral effects and long-term memory, are probably mediated through these complex processes involving regulation of protein phosphorylation and neuronal gene expression. These biochemical and molecular changes lead successively to changes in the function or efficacy of synapses, changes in the way individual neurons process information, and, ultimately, changes in communication among multicellular neural networks.

This chapter illustrates some of the basic mechanisms by which protein phosphorylation and the regulation of neuronal gene expression underlie the extraordinary plasticity evident in both the developing and adult brain. In general, plastic changes mediated through protein phosphorylation do not involve changes in protein synthesis and therefore would be expected to be more rapid in onset, more readily reversible, and shorter lived compared with the plastic changes mediated at the level of the genome.

NEURAL PLASTICITY MEDIATED BY PROTEIN PHOSPHORYLATION

It appears that protein phosphorylation represents the major molecular mechanism underlying neural plasticity. Virtually every type of neuronal protein undergoes phosphorylation and virtually every type of neuronal process is regulated by phosphorylation. Evidence accumulated over the past 20 years has indicated ways in which phosphorylation alters the functional activity of specific proteins and has established the precise mechanisms by which their phosphorylation, in response to neurotransmitters and other extracellular stimuli, mediates short- and long-term effects of those extracellular stimuli on neuronal function (Figure 4–1).

General Aspects of Neuronal Protein Phosphorylation

As discussed in Chapter 2, protein phosphorylation is catalyzed by protein kinases that transfer phosphate groups from ATP to serine, threonine, or tyrosine residues on the target (or substrate) protein. To understand the exact mechanisms by which protein phosphorylation affects neuronal function, it is necessary to understand how it is that the addition of a phosphate group to a protein alters that protein's functional activity.

Phosphorylation of a protein alters that protein's charge (phosphate groups are highly negatively charged), which can then also alter the protein's shape or conformation. When a protein's charge or conformation is altered, it is likely that its intrinsic functional activity will be changed (e.g., the ability of an ion channel to open), or its ability to interact with other molecules will be changed. Phosphorylation has been shown to alter the affinity of certain proteins for other proteins, cofactors (in the case of enzymes), and other small molecules. For example, phosphorylation of tyrosine hydroxylase increases its affinity for its pterin cofactor and thereby increases the rate at which it converts tyrosine to dopa; phosphorylation of the β-adrenergic receptor decreases its affinity for norepinephrine; phosphorylation of certain nuclear proteins alters their ability to initiate transcription of DNA.

The complexity of intracellular regulation is underscored by the now well-established observation that many, perhaps even most, proteins are phosphorylated on more than one amino acid residue by more than one type of protein kinase. This is referred to as "multisite" phosphorylation. Depending on the protein, phosphorylation of different residues can lead to similar or opposite changes in that protein's function. In some cases, the phosphorylation of one residue can even influence the ability of the other residues to undergo phosphorylation.

The phosphorylation of neuronal proteins by more than one protein kinase probably serves to integrate the activities of multiple intracellular pathways to achieve coordinated regulation of cell function. For example, the phosphorylation of tyrosine hydroxylase by cyclic AMP–dependent and Ca^{2+}-dependent protein kinases would enable neurotransmitters that act through the cyclic AMP and Ca^{2+} systems to produce an integrated increase in catecholamine biosynthesis. This example further supports the view that protein phosphorylation is a final common molecular pathway through which multiple extracellular and intracellular signals converge to regulate neuronal function.

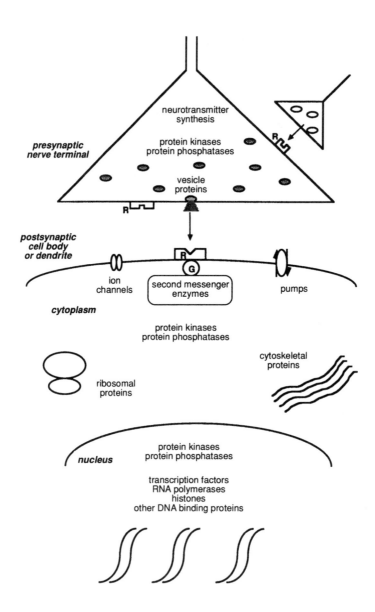

FIGURE 4–1.   Schematic illustration of the types of neuronal proteins regulated by phosphorylation. The figure illustrates that virtually every class of protein, and therefore every type of neural process, is influenced through protein phosphorylation mechanisms. R = receptor. G = G protein.

Examples of Regulation of Neuronal Proteins by Phosphorylation

Regulation of receptors by phosphorylation. For all cases that have been investigated to date, neurotransmitter receptors, both presynaptic and post-synaptic, are regulated by phosphorylation (see Figure 4–1, Table 2–5). In-creasing evidence suggests that phosphorylation alters the functional activity of receptors, for example, their ability to be activated by their endogenous ligand.

In many cases, stimulation of a receptor by its own ligand leads to decreased (or increased) sensitivity of the receptor to subsequent stimulation, processes called "homologous" desensitization (or sensitization) of receptor function. In most cases studied to date this appears to be due to receptor-mediated activation of protein kinases leading to phosphorylation of the receptor. In other cases, a receptor can be phosphorylated by a protein kinase activated by stimulation of another receptor type on the same cell. This could lead to "heterologous" regu-lation of receptor function, whereby receptor phosphorylation induced by one neurotransmitter or second messenger system can influence the responsiveness of a neuron to another neurotransmitter or second messenger system. It is likely that most receptors exhibit both types of regulation and are phosphorylated by more than one protein kinase.

The best-studied example of receptor phosphorylation involves the β-adren-ergic receptor, characterized by Lefkowitz and associates. Activation of the β-adrenergic receptor leads, via coupling with G_s, to activation of adenylate cyclase and to increased levels of cyclic AMP and of activated cyclic AMP–dependent protein kinase, which then appears to phosphorylate the receptor on two serine residues. In addition, the receptor may be phosphorylated on addi-tional serine residues by another protein kinase physically associated with the receptor, termed β-*adrenergic receptor kinase* (or "βark"). This kinase can phosphorylate the receptor only when it is bound to ligand—that is, the binding of ligand to the receptor alters the receptor's conformation such that it is ren-dered a good substrate for the receptor kinase. Phosphorylation of the receptor by either kinase appears to desensitize the receptor to further activation by ad-renergic ligands in vitro and appears to play an important role in producing agonist-mediated desensitization of the receptor in vivo. There is some evi-dence that phosphorylation leads to desensitization by causing the β-receptor to associate with an inhibitory protein that has been called β-arrestin.

In addition to desensitization following stimulation by β-receptor agonists (so-called homologous desensitization), phosphorylation-induced desensitiza-tion of the β-adrenergic receptor can also be stimulated by activation of non-adrenergic receptors that activate the cyclic AMP system and therefore cyclic

AMP–dependent protein kinase (heterologous desensitization). Similar phosphorylation mechanisms have been reported to underlie homologous and heterologous desensitization of other G protein–linked receptors. Notable examples include α-adrenergic and muscarinic cholinergic receptors. As will be seen in Chapter 5, these mechanisms may play a role in the actions of antidepressant drugs.

Regulation of ion channels and pumps by phosphorylation. As with receptors, the functioning of many ion channels can be altered either by direct phosphorylation or by phosphorylation of closely associated proteins (see Table 2–5). In most cases, phosphorylation of the channels modifies their ability to open or close in response to their primary gating mechanism. One example is the L-type voltage-dependent Ca^{2+} channel, the type of channel inhibited by the dihydropyridine Ca^{2+} channel blocker drugs, such as verapamil, used in cardiovascular medicine and occasionally in neuropsychopharmacology. (To date there are four major classes of Ca^{2+} channels that have been identified, termed L, N, T, and P.) When the L-type channel is phosphorylated by cyclic AMP–dependent protein kinase, it is rendered more likely to open in response to membrane depolarization. This mechanism plays an important role in the regulation of cardiac function: the stimulation of β-adrenergic receptors by norepinephrine and epinephrine causes phosphorylation of the channel by increasing levels of cyclic AMP and of activated cyclic AMP–dependent protein kinase. Because the phosphorylated L-type channel opens more, a greater amount of Ca^{2+} enters the cell. In the heart, this mechanism is responsible for catecholamine-induced increases in cardiac rate and contractility. In contrast, the N-type Ca^{2+} channel is found in the presynaptic terminal and is primarily responsible for the Ca^{2+} entry that leads to neurotransmitter release from neurons. It has been hypothesized that phosphorylation of N-type channels in response to neurotransmitters would make them less likely to open and may function as a form of neuromodulation that inhibits neurotransmitter release.

In some cases, phosphorylation of ion channels may represent the primary gating mechanism that determines their opening or closing. One example of such a channel is a slowly depolarizing nonspecific cation channel identified in the rat locus coeruleus. This channel is phosphorylated by cyclic AMP–dependent protein kinase, which appears to initiate opening of the channels. The activity of the channel plays a central role in regulating the spontaneous (i.e., pacemaker) activity of these neurons. Work by Aghajanian and colleagues has shown that the ability of various neurotransmitters (e.g., vasoactive intestinal polypeptide [VIP] or opioid peptides) to regulate the excitability of locus coeruleus neurons is mediated in part through alterations in the activity of this cation channel by cyclic AMP–dependent phosphorylation. Increasing evidence implicates such regulation of locus coeruleus excitability in setting levels of an individual's attention span and vigilance, as well as in mediating behavioral adaptations to stress and opiate addiction (see Chapter 5).

Most types of electrogenic pumps, which maintain stable levels of ions inside and outside of the neuronal membrane, also undergo phosphorylation by second messenger–dependent protein kinases. These include the Na^+-K^+ ATPase and the Ca^{2+}-Mg^{2+} ATPase pumps. Phosphorylation and regulation of the activity of the Na^+-K^+ ATPase pump would alter the rate at which the normal distribution of ions can be restored after a train of action potentials. This would be expected to alter the excitability of the neurons. Such a mechanism has recently been shown to operate in the brain, where dopamine, via regulation of cyclic AMP–dependent protein phosphorylation, regulates activity of the Na^+-K^+ ATPase pump in striatal neurons. Through this mechanism, dopamine can produce relatively long-lasting changes in striatal neuronal excitability. This mechanism may be significant for extrapyramidal regulation of movement under normal conditions and the extrapyramidal side effects of antipsychotic drugs. Similarly, phosphorylation and regulation of the activity of the Ca^{2+}-Mg^{2+} ATPase pump would alter the excitability of neurons by influencing the ability of neurons to maintain the normal (low) levels of intracellular free Ca^{2+} and to maintain healthy stores of Ca^{2+} in intracellular organelles.

Regulation of intracellular messenger pathways by phosphorylation. Most of the protein components of intracellular messenger systems are themselves phosphoproteins (i.e., substrates for protein kinases; see Table 2–5). This permits extraordinarily complex cross-talk between signaling pathways, allowing cells to coordinate their responses to environmental stimuli. Virtually every type of G protein has been reported to undergo phosphorylation by various protein kinases.

Proteins that control the synthesis of the cyclic nucleotide second messengers (adenylate cyclase and guanylate cyclase), as well as the degradation of cyclic nucleotides (phosphodiesterases), are regulated by phosphorylation. Similarly, proteins that lead to increases in intracellular Ca^{2+} or phosphatidylinositol turnover (e.g., phospholipase C, Ca^{2+} channels, the inositol triphosphate [IP_3] receptor) and proteins that decrease Ca^{2+} levels (e.g., the Ca^{2+}-Mg^{2+} ATPase pump) are regulated by phosphorylation. Moreover, phospholipase A_2, which generates arachidonic acid metabolites (e.g., prostaglandins) that modulate cyclic nucleotide and Ca^{2+} levels, is also subject to phosphorylation. Many protein kinases are themselves phosphorylated and regulated by other protein kinases, and protein phosphatase type 1 (which removes phosphate groups) is regulated by protein phosphatase inhibitor proteins, which themselves are regulated by phosphorylation.

In addition, most, and possibly all, protein kinases undergo autophosphorylation, whereby they phosphorylate themselves. In most cases, such autophosphorylation appears to facilitate activation of the enzyme. For example, autophosphorylation of Ca^{2+}/calmodulin–dependent protein kinase II renders the protein kinase independent of Ca^{2+}. This means that the enzyme, activated originally in response to elevated levels of cellular Ca^{2+}, remains active after Ca^{2+} levels have returned to baseline. By this mechanism, neurotransmitters that activate Ca^{2+}/calmodulin–dependent protein kinase II can produce relatively long-lived alterations in neuronal function. In other cases, autophosphorylation may be a necessary event in the activation of the protein kinase. Defects in autophosphorylation of the insulin receptor (which, in addition to its insulin binding site, has protein tyrosine kinase activity) underlie peripheral insulin resistance seen in some families with diabetes mellitus.

It is clear from the above discussion that each second messenger system in the brain influences all the others. This means that although the systems are drawn as distinct pathways in Figures 2–6, 2–8, and 2–9, they do not operate as distinct pathways, but operate instead as a complex web of interacting pathways. Thus, any time a neurotransmitter produces its primary effect on one second messenger system, all other systems will also be influenced eventually, with such interactions mediated for the most part through protein phosphorylation. For example, a neurotransmitter that produces its primary effect on the cyclic AMP system would be expected to influence the Ca^{2+} and phosphatidylinositol systems through the phosphorylation, by cyclic AMP–dependent protein kinase, of G proteins, phospholipases, Ca^{2+} channels, Ca^{2+}-dependent protein kinases, the IP_3 receptor, and common substrate proteins for cyclic AMP–dependent and Ca^{2+}-dependent protein kinases.

Regulation of neurotransmitter metabolism by phosphorylation. Neurotransmitter synthetic enzymes are known to be regulated by phosphorylation (see Table 2–5). For example, as discussed in Chapter 3, tyrosine hydroxylase, the rate-limiting enzyme in the synthesis of the catecholamine neurotransmitters, is phosphorylated and activated by cyclic AMP–dependent protein kinase, Ca^{2+}/calmodulin–dependent protein kinase, protein kinase C, and other protein kinases. Phosphorylation appears to have its major affect on tyrosine hydroxylase by increasing the affinity of the enzyme for its pterin cofactor (which would make the enzyme more active at the subsaturating concentrations of cofactor found physiologically). In addition, when tyrosine hydroxylase is phosphorylated, it is less inhibitable by the end products of catecholamine biosynthesis (dopamine and norepinephrine). Such phosphorylation of the enzyme has been shown to mediate the ability of many types of neurotransmitters (acting through the cyclic AMP and/or Ca^{2+} systems) to rapidly increase tyrosine hydroxylase activity and, as a result, the capacity of catecholaminergic neurons to synthesize their neurotransmitter. This provides a critical homeostatic control mechanism that enables catecholaminergic neurons to alter their functional activity in response to a variety of synaptic inputs.

Similarly, tryptophan hydroxylase, the rate-limiting enzyme in the synthesis of serotonin, is phosphorylated and regulated by Ca^{2+}/calmodulin–dependent protein kinase II. Such phosphorylation presumably mediates the ability of neurotransmitters that activate the Ca^{2+} system to regulate serotonin biosynthesis in vivo.

Regulation of neurotransmitter release by phosphorylation. As described in the discussion on ion channels above, regulation of Ca^{2+} channel phosphorylation can alter the entry of Ca^{2+} into nerve terminals and thereby the release of neurotransmitter from those terminals. Regulation of other types of channels could similarly alter neurotransmitter release by indirectly influencing the amount of Ca^{2+} that enters the terminals during an action potential. However, there are additional important mechanisms by which neurotransmitter release is regulated in the brain independent of ion channel phosphorylation. These appear to involve the phosphorylation of a variety of synaptic vesicle–associated proteins (see Table 2–5). Such regulation of neurotransmitter release is an important mechanism by which behavioral stimuli and psychotropic drugs modulate the strength of specific synaptic connections in the brain.

The best-studied synaptic vesicle–associated phosphoproteins are the synapsins, first discovered by Greengard and associates in the early 1970s. The synapsins comprise a family of phosphoproteins present in most synaptic terminals in the brain that are phosphorylated by cyclic AMP–dependent protein kinase and by Ca^{2+}/calmodulin–dependent protein kinases I and II.

Synapsin phosphorylation increases the amount of neurotransmitter released from nerve terminals in response to physiological stimuli. Phosphorylation of synapsins appears to augment neurotransmitter release by altering their binding affinity for synaptic vesicles and other cytoskeletal proteins. Such changes in synapsin binding affinities are thought to regulate synaptic vesicle traffic within nerve terminals and, possibly, the process of exocytosis.

Phosphorylation of the synapsins is regulated by a number of neurotransmitters that influence cyclic AMP or Ca^{2+} levels in nerve terminals and appears to mediate the ability of these neurotransmitters to produce relatively long-lasting changes in the functional activity of those terminals. Phosphorylation of the synapsins also occurs in response to action potentials and probably represents one mechanism underlying posttetanic potentiation, or PTP. PTP, a phenomenon originally described decades ago, occurs in most types of nerve terminals, where a brief series of nerve impulses (referred to as a *tetanus*) increases the amount of neurotransmitter released by the terminals in response to a subsequent nerve impulse.

Regulation of neuronal growth and differentiation by phosphorylation. Protein phosphorylation also plays a critical role in cell growth, differentiation, and movement, although the details of the mechanisms remain obscure. Virtually all known cytoskeletal and contractile proteins are heavily phosphorylated by a number of protein kinases, and, in many cases, their functional activity is known to be altered on phosphorylation (Table 2–5). Specific types of protein kinases are induced in cells, including neurons, at precise points during the cell cycle. Similarly, specific types of protein kinases and substrate proteins are expressed in the brain at particular stages during development and differentiation. Neural cell adhesion molecules and proteins expressed specifically in axonal growth cones (the leading tips of growing axons), both of which are important for cell-cell interactions in the brain and the formation of synaptic connections, are also regulated by phosphorylation.

Regulation of gene expression by phosphorylation. In recent years, it has become clear that protein phosphorylation also plays a fundamental role in the regulation of neuronal gene expression, in a sense the ultimate end point of signal transduction in the brain. Such regulation appears to be achieved through the phosphorylation of a subset of the proteins that regulate transcription, including transcription factors, RNA polymerase, and a variety of other nonhistone and histone nuclear proteins (see Table 2–5 and Figures 4–2 and 4–3).

TRANSSYNAPTIC REGULATION OF GENE EXPRESSION

As mentioned above, regulation of neural gene expression by neurotransmitters, which occurs continually to replace proteins that are turning over and to adapt brain function to myriad environmental inputs, can, under certain circumstances, produce long-lasting alterations in virtually all aspects of a neuron's functioning—via altered levels of neurotransmitter-synthesizing enzymes, peptide neurotransmitters, receptors, ion channels, signal transduction proteins, cytoskeletal components within the cells, and other critical neural proteins.

Gene expression in the brain can be activated by normal physiological processes, by drugs, and by experience. Afferent sensory data activate particular neural networks in the brain, which in turn activate neurons involved in higher-order processing. Within each of these cells, the generation of action potentials and the activation of second messenger systems would be expected to alter the rate of expression of specific genes and as a result the expression of multiple types of neuronal proteins. Altered levels of these proteins would produce characteristic changes in the way the affected neurons process subsequent synaptic information. Such mechanisms probably underlie many of the long-term consequences of sensory input, including behavioral stimuli, on brain function (e.g., types of learning). It is likely that most psychotropic drugs influence neuronal gene expression via similar synaptic events, although some drugs may influence neuronal gene expression via direct effects on intracellular messengers (see Chapter 5).

The process by which activity in one neuron regulates gene expression in another neuron is referred to as *transsynaptic regulation of gene expression,* a term first coined by Costa and colleagues close to 20 years ago. We now know that a class of proteins termed *transcription factors* play a central role in transsynaptic regulation of neural gene expression.

Transcription Factors

As discussed in Chapter 1, transcription factors are proteins that bind to specific DNA sequences in the regulatory regions of genes. The binding of transcription factors to these regulatory sequences increases or decreases the rate at which those genes are transcribed. Many types of transcription factors are known; these can be categorized into families of related proteins based on their structure and function. Some well-known families of transcription factors that may play important roles in neuronal adaptation are given in Table 4–1.

Some transcription factors are designated by functional features (e.g., the steroid receptors); others are designated by structural features. *Leucine zippers* are protein domains found in several families of transcription factors that permit dimerization of these factors. *Zinc fingers* are structural regions of other transcription factors (regions rich in cysteines surrounding a zinc ion) that are involved in binding of the protein to the DNA. The *fos/jun* family and *zif*268 are regulated as immediate early genes.

There are two general mechanisms by which transcription factors mediate transsynaptic regulation of gene expression (Figures 4–2 and 4–3). One mechanism involves neurotransmitter receptor–mediated activation of a transcription factor that preexists within the neuron (i.e., synthesis of the factor is a constitutive feature of that type of neuron and is not dependent on stimulation). Activation of preexisting factors can be achieved by phosphorylation (or dephosphorylation) of the transcription factor or by its translocation into the nucleus.

The other mechanism requires de novo synthesis of a transcription factor in response to stimulation of the cell; the newly synthesized factor can then activate or repress other genes. The first mechanism occurs more rapidly than the second and partly explains the widely different time courses observed for transsynaptic regulation of gene expression. Thus, some neurotransmitter receptor–stimulated changes in gene expression occur within minutes, whereas others may require many hours. We will illustrate mechanisms underlying the transsynaptic regulation of gene expression by considering specific examples in the nervous system.

CREB proteins.   Cyclic AMP response element binding (CREB) proteins are a family of related proteins that bind to a particular DNA sequence termed the *cyclic AMP response element,* or CRE (containing the nucleotides TGACGTCA or a closely related sequence). CREB proteins play a major role in mediating the effects of cyclic AMP, and of those neurotransmitters that act through cyclic AMP, on gene expression. A large and increasing number of genes have been shown to contain CREs; some examples, discussed below, are the genes for Fos,

---

FIGURE 4–2 *(at right).*   **Schematic illustration of the intracellular pathways underlying transsynaptic regulation of gene expression, Part I.** Activation of neurotransmitter or hormone receptors leads to the activation of specific second messenger and protein phosphorylation systems, which produce multiple effects on neuronal function through the phosphorylation of numerous types of substrate proteins, as described in the text.

Among the effects of these intracellular systems on neuronal function is the regulation of gene expression. This can be accomplished by two basic types of mechanisms. In one case, transcription factors, already in the nucleus, are phosphorylated directly by protein kinases; this alters their transcriptional activity and thereby leads to alterations in the expression of numerous target genes. Transcription factors that function in this manner include the CREB-like proteins, which can be viewed as "third messengers" in that they are the first proteins to be phosphorylated in this pathway. Among the target genes for the CREB-like transcription factors are those for other transcription factors, for example, Fos and related immediate early gene products. Increased expression of Fos and related transcription factors then leads to alterations in the expression of specific target genes. Fos-like proteins can be viewed as "fourth messengers," although they are sometimes referred to in the literature as third messengers. Another class of transcription factors, the steroid hormone receptors, are not shown.

IP_3 = inositol triphosphate.

proenkephalin, somatostatin, tyrosine hydroxylase, and VIP.

The primary mechanism by which CREB proteins are regulated, and thereby mediate transsynaptic changes in gene expression, is through phosphorylation by cyclic AMP–dependent protein kinase. CREB proteins appear to be constitutively synthesized so that they exist in neurons at roughly constant levels. According to one possible scheme, CREB proteins are localized under resting conditions to the nucleus, where they are bound to CREs without considerable transcriptional activity. Phosphorylation of CREB proteins activates their transcriptional activity, apparently by stimulating their ability to interact with some component of the polymerase II complex. An alternative scheme is that phos-

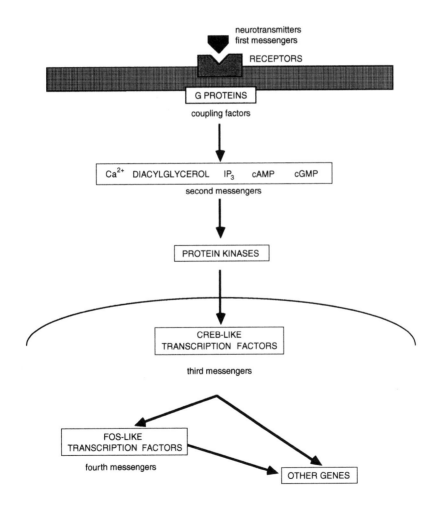

phorylation of some CREB proteins stimulates their transcriptional activity also by enhancing their binding affinity for the CRE on the DNA.

The mechanism by which neurotransmitters that increase cyclic AMP levels would regulate gene expression via CREB proteins is shown in Figures 4–2 and

FIGURE 4–3 *(at right).*   **Schematic illustration of the intracellular pathways under-lying transsynaptic regulation of gene expression, Part II.** The figure begins to illustrate the potential complexity of the actual mechanisms that underlie the more simplified model of transsynaptic regulation of gene expression shown in Figure 4–2.

Three genes are shown in the figure: the genes that code for hypothetical transcription factors 1 and 2 (TF-1 and TF-2) and the gene that codes for some cellular protein (Protein X). Each gene contains a coding region, from which mRNA is synthesized in the nucleus by the enzyme RNA polymerase II. The mRNAs for all proteins must then be transported into the cytoplasm, where proteins are synthesized by ribosomes. Each gene also contains a promoter region that possesses sequences of DNA or response elements (indicated in the figure by the irregular shapes along the promoter) that recognize specific types of transcription factors. The expression of a particular gene, as shown for Protein X, is determined typically by the activity of multiple types of transcription factors interacting with multiple response elements in that gene's promoter region. The figure also illustrates that some transcription factors, as shown for TF-2, regulate their own expression. In addition, the expression of transcription factors can be regulated by other transcription factors, as shown for TF-1, expression of which is also regulated by TF-2. Both mechanisms appear to operate for the transcription factor Fos, expression of which is known to be regulated by itself and by a number of other transcription factors, for example, CREB (see Figure 4–2).

The figure illustrates two general cellular locations for transcription factor phosphorylation. Some transcription factors, as shown for TF-1, are phosphorylated in the cytoplasm by cytoplasmic protein kinases activated in response to specific neurotransmitter or second messenger signals. Such phosphorylated transcription factors are translocated to the nucleus, where they interact with a specific response element in a target gene's promoter region. Examples of transcription factors that appear to undergo such cytoplasmic phosphorylation are steroid hormone receptors. Phosphorylation of the receptors may regulate the ability of the steroid hormone to bind to the receptor and promote its translocation into the nucleus and/or the ability of the receptor to bind to its response element. In either case, cytoplasmic phosphorylation of the steroid receptors would alter their physiological activity and thereby mediate some of the effects of the original neurotransmitter signal on neuronal gene expression.

Other transcription factors, as shown for TF-2, after cytoplasmic synthesis and translocation to the nucleus, are phosphorylated by nuclear protein kinases activated in response to specific neurotransmitter or second messenger signals. Examples of transcription factors that appear to undergo such nuclear phosphorylation are the CREB proteins. Phosphorylation of CREB protein apparently regulates its ability to interact with some component of the RNA polymerase II complex. Such phosphorylation increases CREB protein's transcriptional activity and thereby mediates some of the effects of the original neurotransmitter signal on neuronal gene expression.

R = receptor. G = G protein. P = phosphate.

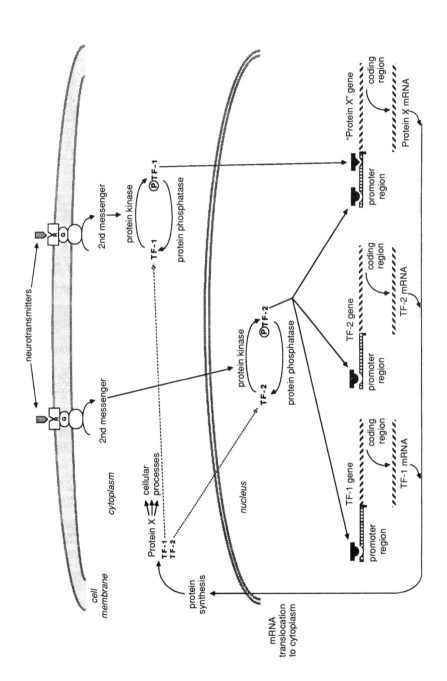

4–3. Neurotransmitter receptor stimulation would increase levels of cyclic AMP and of activated cyclic AMP–dependent protein kinase. Activated protein kinase (i.e., free catalytic subunits of the enzyme) would then be translocated into the nucleus, where they would phosphorylate and activate CREB protein. Phosphorylation of CREB protein would, in turn, activate the expression of genes that contain CREB protein bound to their promoter regions.

In actuality, regulation of CREB proteins is far more complicated than described above. The CREB family of proteins not only mediate some of the actions of cyclic AMP on gene expression, but they also appear to mediate some of the effects of Ca^{2+}, which might enter cells as a result of depolarization. Indirect evidence suggests that cyclic AMP–dependent and Ca^{2+}/calmodulin–dependent protein kinases phosphorylate certain form(s) of CREB on distinct residues and that phosphorylation of the protein by both enzymes results in its synergistic activation.

In addition, CREB is part of a family of related transcription factors, different members of which may have maximal binding affinities to slightly different response elements. Moreover, these different forms may not all confer second messenger responsiveness on the gene to which they bind. Different CREB-like proteins may be expressed at different levels in different neuronal cell types throughout the brain. Finally, although it is generally thought that the total amounts of CREB proteins are not regulated in the nervous system, this possibility has not been ruled out.

Immediate early genes. Immediate early genes (IEGs) are so named because their transcription is activated rapidly (within minutes) and transiently, and without the requirement for new protein synthesis. The terminology was

---

TABLE 4–1.　　Transcription factors in the brain

Leucine zipper proteins
  CREB/ATF family
  Fos/Jun family, e.g.,
    c-Fos
    Fos-related antigens (FRAs)
    c-Jun
    JunB
    JunD

Zinc finger proteins
  e.g., Zif268

Steroid/thyroid hormone/retinoic acid receptor family

---

developed initially to describe viral genes that are activated "immediately" (within minutes) on infection of eukaryotic cells. Viral IEGs encode transcription factors that are needed to activate viral "late" gene expression. The terminology has been extended to cellular (i.e., nonviral) genes; cellular IEGs often, but not always, encode transcription factors. Cellular IEGs that have been shown to be rapidly activated in neurons in response to neurotransmitters and drugs include members of the related *fos* and *jun* families and *zif*268 (Table 4–1).

Another frequently used terminology also applies to certain IEGs. Many IEGs, including *fos* and *jun*, are also found in certain viruses in altered (mutated) forms. The forms of these genes carried by viruses have often lost regulatory mechanisms and, because they are transcription factors, may activate expression of target genes to vast excess. Not surprisingly, this may lead to malignant transformation of susceptible cells. These viral forms, known as v-*fos* and v-*jun*, are described as oncogenes. The regulated cellular forms, known as c-*fos* and c-*jun*, are often referred to as proto-oncogenes. By convention, viral oncogenes have the prefix "v-" and cellular proto-oncogenes have the prefix "c-." Oncogenes are written in lowercase italic (e.g., *fos*), and their protein products begin with an uppercase letter, with no italic (e.g., Fos). To complicate matters further, not all oncogenes are IEGs. Many contain dysregulated forms of other genes whose products (e.g., growth factor receptors or signal transduction proteins such as G proteins and protein kinases) also cause inappropriate regulation of cell growth.

In many cases, the protein products of cellular IEGs may interact with themselves or one another to form a potentially large number of transcriptionally active homodimers (two molecules of the same protein) or heterodimers (two different molecules) that bind to specific regulatory elements within genes. The well-studied heterodimeric IEG pair composed of Fos and Jun binds to a DNA sequence (TGACTCA) termed the activator protein-1 (AP-1) site. Dimers composed of different members of the Fos and Jun families may have differences in their binding properties as well as in other characteristics.

There is now a great deal of evidence to show that the primary mechanism by which *fos* itself is regulated, and thereby mediates transsynaptic changes in expression of other genes, is at the transcriptional level (see Figures 4–2 and 4–3). Fos is present in most neurons at barely detectable levels under resting conditions, but expression of its gene can be induced dramatically in response to various stimuli, including neuronal depolarization. The newly synthesized *fos* messenger RNA (mRNA) is then translocated to the cytoplasm where it is translated into new Fos protein. Fos protein, in turn, is translocated back to the nucleus where, in conjunction with a member of the Jun family, it binds to AP-1 sites on the promoter regions of numerous target genes and regulates their expression. Identification of neural target genes for cellular IEGs is currently a focus of much research. Two possibilities include the genes for proenkephalin and tyrosine hydroxylase (see below).

The precise intracellular mechanisms by which extracellular stimuli induce Fos expression are becoming increasingly well understood. Stimuli that depolarize neurons (e.g., seizure activity and glutamate) appear to induce Fos through a Ca^{2+}-dependent mechanism that involves the phosphorylation by a Ca^{2+}/calmodulin–dependent protein kinase of a CREB protein that is already present in the cell and bound to a CRE in the *fos* gene promoter. Phosphorylation of a CREB protein, as outlined above, activates its transcriptional activity and leads to increased *fos* mRNA expression. Stimuli that increase cyclic AMP levels in neurons, without an increase in Ca^{2+} levels (e.g., VIP, corticotropin-releasing factor, norepinephrine at β-adrenergic receptors, dopamine at D_1 receptors), can also induce Fos, apparently through the phosphorylation by cyclic AMP–dependent protein kinase of the same or a related CREB protein. Such induction of Fos could then mediate some of the effects of the original extracellular stimuli, acting through the Ca^{2+} or cyclic AMP systems, on the expression of specific target genes.

The finding that depolarizing stimuli induce Fos has led to the suggestion by Morgan and Curran and their colleagues that Fos can be used as a way to map neuronal activity in the brain. Indeed, Fos has been shown to be induced in specific regions of the nervous system by many stimuli associated with increased neural activity. Some examples include induction of Fos in the dorsal horn of the spinal cord by physiological stimulation of primary sensory neurons, in motor and sensory thalamic nuclei by stimulation of the sensory cortex, in supraoptic and paraventricular nuclei by water deprivation, and in numerous brain regions by acute and chronic opiate and cocaine administration, as well as in response to a number of other psychotropic drug treatments.

Induction of other IEGs is also observed in the nervous system in response to many of these same stimuli. Thus, c-Jun, JunB, and Zif268, as well as Fos-like proteins referred to as Fos-related antigens (FRAs), are induced under many of the same conditions as those observed for Fos. However, important differences exist in the time courses of their induction. Zif268 and c-Fos appear to be the most rapidly and transiently induced, with protein levels maximally elevated within 2 hours after an appropriate stimulus and returned to normal within 6 hours. Other proteins may be induced with slightly slower time courses and may remain elevated for considerably longer times.

The activation of IEG products such as Fos in response to a large number of stimuli raises the question of how specificity of response is achieved. First, specificity is partly achieved by the particular neural circuitry involved; that is, Fos and the other proteins are induced only along those particular neural pathways that are activated in response to some stimulus.

Second, specificity is achieved by specialization within neuronal cell types. For example, in particular cell types, not every gene that contains an appropriate binding site, for example, an AP-1 site, to which Fos can bind is in a chromatin configuration that permits access to Fos-containing complexes.

Third, individual transcription factors generally cannot act alone to induce or repress the expression of a given gene. Multiple types of transcription factors, binding to distinct regulatory elements within a gene's promoter region, must often act in concert to produce significant effects on gene expression.

Fourth, as alluded to above, protein products of many IEGs including Fos can only bind DNA with high affinity after binding to other transcription factors to form heterodimers. Such interactions are well exemplified by c-Fos and c-Jun. By itself, c-Fos is unable to bind DNA with high affinity. c-Jun homodimers can bind DNA, but do so with relatively low affinity. However, Fos-Jun heterodimers bind to the AP-1 site with high affinity to regulate transcription. In contrast, heterodimers of Fos and JunB appear to be relatively inactive and may therefore serve an inhibitory function. Because there appear to be many members of the *fos* and *jun* families, complex regulatory schemes can readily be imagined by which a great deal of specificity in regulating cellular genes can be attained.

Although the primary mechanism by which *fos* and the other IEGs are regulated appears to be at the level of their transcription, the proteins are probably also regulated by phosphorylation. For example, Fos is known to be heavily phosphorylated on a number of closely spaced serine residues in the carboxy terminal region of the protein by cyclic AMP–dependent and Ca^{2+}/calmodulin–dependent protein kinases and by protein kinase C. Fos phosphorylation appears to be a critical regulatory mechanism for the protein: the difference between normal cellular *fos* and its viral counterpart (which is oncogenic) is a frameshift mutation that deletes the serine residues from the viral protein. Interestingly, a recent report suggests that phosphorylation of Fos renders the protein able to suppress its own transcription, thereby providing key regulatory feedback control on the expression of this transcription factor.

Protein kinase C also plays an important role in the functional activity of the IEG products. In fact, the AP-1 DNA sequence was first identified as the response element that confers sensitivity of a gene to transcriptional regulation by protein kinase C or agents, such as phorbol esters, that activate protein kinase C. However, the mechanism by which protein kinase C regulates the functional activity of Fos-Jun heterodimers remains unknown. Fos or Jun may be directly phosphorylated and activated by protein kinase C. It is also possible that some other protein that interacts with Fos-Jun complexes, and that is involved in transcriptional machinery, is phosphorylated by this protein kinase.

Steroid and thyroid hormone receptors.   The primary mechanism by which steroid and thyroid hormones regulate cell function is by increasing or decreasing the expression of specific sets of genes in target tissues, including brain tissue. Unlike most hormones and neurotransmitters that bind to extracellular receptors, steroid and thyroid hormones bind to a family of related cytoplasmic receptors. This binding leads to the translocation of the receptor-hormone complexes into the nucleus, where the complexes bind to specific DNA sequences (e.g., glucocorticoid response elements) in target genes and thereby alter the rates at which those genes are transcribed. Thus, steroid and thyroid hormone receptors represent a class of proteins that function as ligand-regulated transcription factors. A major focus of current research is to identify the target genes for these hormones in the brain.

Although the primary mechanism by which the transcriptional activity of steroid and thyroid hormone receptors is regulated is through their ligand binding and consequent nuclear translocation, the receptors are also regulated in vivo at transcriptional and posttranslational levels. Such regulation probably modulates the physiological responsiveness of the receptors. The total amount of the receptors expressed in specific target tissues can be altered by various hormonal and drug treatments, including in vivo treatment of animals with antidepressant medications. Steroid and thyroid hormone receptors are also known to be phosphorylated by cyclic AMP–dependent and Ca^{2+}-dependent protein kinases and by protein tyrosine kinases. The physiological role of receptor phosphorylation remains unknown, but it could alter the affinity of the receptors for their ligands, their translocation into the nucleus, and/or their binding to their DNA response elements.

Regulation of Proenkephalin and Tyrosine Hydroxylase: Model Systems for the Study of Neural Gene Expression

Proenkephalin.   Proenkephalin is the peptide precursor of the enkephalins—endogenous opioid peptides that serve neurotransmitter roles in the nervous system (see Chapter 3). Many investigators have shown that both the synthesis and release of enkephalins are regulated by synaptic activity. The most important control point for proenkephalin synthesis appears to be at the level of transcription.

The influence of first and second messengers on proenkephalin gene expression has been examined in great detail. Proenkephalin mRNA levels have been shown to be increased by a number of stimuli, including increased neural activity and various neurotransmitters and drugs. These first messengers appear to regulate the expression of proenkephalin through the activation of cyclic AMP–

dependent protein kinase, protein kinase C, or other Ca^{2+}-dependent protein kinases. The specific transcription factors that mediate this regulation appear to be members of the Fos and Jun families.

One example of the physiological regulation of proenkephalin gene expression is insulin shock, a rat model of stress that stimulates the adrenal medulla by increasing impulse traffic in the splanchnic nerve. Increased nicotinic cholinergic stimulation of the adrenal medulla leads to marked increases in levels of mRNA encoding proenkephalin (and also other neurotransmitter-related genes, such as that for tyrosine hydroxylase). Regulation of proenkephalin mRNA levels has also been shown to occur in the brain. Administration of the antipsychotic drug haloperidol or of lithium increases levels of proenkephalin mRNA in rat striatum. Chronic stress and chronic opiate administration also regulate proenkephalin mRNA expression in specific brain regions. In addition, seizures induced by electrical or chemical means (e.g., by pentylenetetrazol) produce striking increases in expression of proenkephalin in dentate granule cells in the hippocampus. This is particularly interesting because seizures have also been shown to induce a number of IEGs, including c-*fos* and c-*jun,* in these hippocampal neurons. Recall that Fos and Jun proteins can form heterodimers that bind to DNA at AP-1 binding sites to activate gene expression. Because the proenkephalin gene contains an AP-1 site, some investigators have argued that activation of c-*fos* and c-*jun* by seizures causes the subsequent activation of proenkephalin gene expression in those cells. Further work is needed to confirm the validity of this mechanism. Nevertheless, it provides a good model for how activation of cellular IEGs might contribute to subsequent changes in the expression of specific neural genes (see Figure 4–2).

It should be pointed out that such models of the regulation of gene expression by seizures may eventually contribute to the generation of specific mechanistic hypotheses of how electroconvulsive therapy produces pervasive changes in affective states and how complex partial seizures might produce long-term changes in the mood and cognition of patients afflicted with this seizure disorder.

Tyrosine hydroxylase. Tyrosine hydroxylase also serves as a good model for transsynaptic regulation of gene expression. The expression of tyrosine hydroxylase has been shown to be regulated by cholinergic stimulation in adrenal medulla, peripheral sympathetic neurons, and cultured pheochromocytoma cells. Regulation also occurs in central catecholaminergic neurons in response to a variety of stimuli. Neural activity appears to be one of the primary signals that determines the level of enzyme expression in these various cell types, although other mechanisms may also be involved, as will be discussed below. Examples of stimuli that alter tyrosine hydroxylase expression in central neurons are acute and chronic stress and numerous chronic drug treatments, including morphine, cocaine, reserpine, and antidepressant drugs. Altered levels of tyrosine hydroxylase expression presumably represent an adaptive response of catecholaminergic neurons that enables the cells to function at an altered rate of neural activity.

Considerable progress has been made in recent years in defining the precise intracellular mechanisms by which extracellular stimuli alter the expression of tyrosine hydroxylase. The gene that codes tyrosine hydroxylase has been cloned, and specific response elements have been identified in the promoter region of the gene. The promoter contains a CRE and an AP-1–like binding site. Information available to date suggests several schemes by which physiological and pharmacological stimuli could regulate tyrosine hydroxylase at the level of gene expression.

First, enzyme expression induced by increased neural activity (depolarization) appears to be mediated via the Ca^{2+}-dependent phosphorylation of a CREB protein bound to the CRE. Second, such enzyme induction could hypothetically also be mediated via an indirect mechanism in which neural activity induces Fos and/or related IEGs that would then activate enzyme expression by binding to the AP-1 site. Third, tyrosine hydroxylase gene expression induced in response to neurotransmitters that increase neuronal levels of cyclic AMP could be mediated via activation of cyclic AMP–dependent protein kinase and the phosphorylation of CREB protein. Fourth, enzyme expression is induced in some cell types by glucocorticoids, an effect mediated presumably via hormone binding to cytoplasmic receptors that would then translocate to the nucleus and bind to as yet unidentified glucocorticoid response elements. Future work will be directed at defining which of these mechanisms operates in the central nervous system in response to various behavioral and pharmacological stimuli known to regulate tyrosine hydroxylase in vivo.

Nontranscriptional Control of Protein Expression

Up to this point, we have focused on alterations in the levels of neuronal proteins mediated at the level of gene transcription. However, the total amount of a protein can also be altered at a number of other levels. For example, the level of a protein would change, despite a constant rate of transcription, if its mRNA were degraded or translated at a different rate. Similarly, the level of a protein would change, despite a constant rate of mRNA translation, if it were degraded at a different rate. In recent years, it has become apparent that changes in mRNA and protein stability probably contribute to neurotransmitter-induced changes in protein levels. The stability and translatability of specific mRNAs have been shown to be regulated by cyclic AMP– and Ca^{2+}-dependent mechanisms, and a family of proteases (enzymes that degrade proteins) have been shown to be specifically activated by increases in cellular Ca^{2+} levels. The multitude of mechanisms by which total amounts of proteins can be regulated in a neuron (transcriptionally, posttranscriptionally, and posttranslationally) underscores the complex mechanisms utilized by neurons to maintain their homeostatic balance.

MOLECULAR BASIS OF LEARNING AND MEMORY

Understanding how the brain learns and stores memories is a central goal of neurobiology. The neurotransmitter- and drug-induced changes in protein phosphorylation and gene expression discussed in the preceding sections of this chapter represent forms of molecular "memory" within individual neurons. In all likelihood, learning and memory at the level of the whole brain are mediated by complex accumulations of these basic types of changes to produce alterations in the function or efficacy of synapses within particular neural systems. Changes in synaptic efficacy may be due to altered patterns of neurotransmitter release by the presynaptic neuron or changes in the effect of neurotransmitter on the postsynaptic cell. Because alterations in protein phosphorylation tend to be more readily reversible than alterations in gene expression, it is often hypothesized that regulation of the phosphorylation state of particular proteins may underlie short-term memory, whereas changes in gene expression leading to new protein synthesis may be required for longer-term memory. A goal of current research is to relate specific alterations in the phosphorylation or expression of proteins to specific behavioral phenomena.

Two candidate mechanisms of memory have received particular attention, one of which, long-term potentiation, has been documented in the vertebrate brain. The other, a model of presynaptic facilitation, has been studied in the invertebrate nervous system, most notably in the marine mollusk *Aplysia*. These mechanisms are described below.

Long-Term Potentiation

Long-term potentiation (LTP) has received considerable attention as a potential mechanism of memory in the mammalian brain. Evidence accumulating since the 1950s has established that the hippocampus is required for the initial storage of long-term memories. Damage to the hippocampus, especially if it is bilateral, produces an amnesia syndrome in which memories obtained during the preceding several weeks are lost and new long-term memories cannot be formed. Normally memories are consolidated over days to weeks (by a process that is not understood) for storage outside the hippocampus, presumably in association areas of the cerebral cortex, so that hippocampal damage does not affect older memories.

Not only is the hippocampus the initial site required for long-term memories, it has also been known for two decades to be a site for a kind of long-term synaptic facilitation called *long-term potentiation*. LTP has been shown to occur by different mechanisms at the three major synaptic pathways in the hippocampus: 1) the perforant pathway, which synapses on the dentate gyrus granule cells, 2) the pathway by which these granule cells send their axons (called mossy fibers) to synapse on the pyramidal cells in region CA_3 of the hippocampus, and 3) the pathway by which pyramidal cells in CA_3 send their axons (called Schaeffer collaterals) to synapse on pyramidal cells of the CA_1 region. LTP occurring at synapses within area CA_1 of the hippocampus represents the most widely studied form of activity-dependent synaptic plasticity in the mammalian nervous system.

LTP can be induced experimentally in vivo in area CA_1 of the hippocampus by stimulating the presynaptic fibers (the Schaeffer collateral pathway) with a brief train of high-frequency electrical impulses (often referred to as a *tetanus*), resembling impulse trains that can occur physiologically. The result of the tetanus is a marked and long-lasting enhancement in the functional responsiveness of postsynaptic cells to subsequent stimulation (i.e., depolarizing stimuli produce a much larger synaptic current after induction of LTP than before). LTP induced in vivo in the CA_1 region of the hippocampus can last for weeks. Synapses in the CA_1 region that can express LTP utilize glutamate as their neurotransmitter. As described in Chapter 3, glutamate receptor types (named for their selective agonists) include *N*-methyl-D-aspartate (NMDA) receptors and two types of non-NMDA receptors (kainate and α-amino-3-hydroxy-5-methyl-4-isoxalone propionic acid [AMPA]). Activation of kainate and AMPA receptors causes increased permeability to Na^+ and, hence, depolarization of the postsynaptic neuron. NMDA receptors can permit entry of both Na^+ and Ca^{2+}, but can only be activated by glutamate if the postsynaptic cell is also depolarized. As described in Chapter 3, depolarization is required to relieve a block of the NMDA receptor channel by Mg^{2+}. Thus, the NMDA receptor channel is both ligand and voltage gated.

In hippocampal CA_1 neurons, LTP can only be activated if Ca^{2+} enters the postsynaptic neuron via NMDA receptor channels. Compounds that selectively block the glutamate binding site on NMDA receptors (e.g., D-2-amino-5-phosphonovalerate [AP5, or APV]) or that block the NMDA receptor channel (e.g.,

MK-801, recently renamed dizocilpine) block the initiation of LTP. Because Ca^{2+} entry into the postsynaptic cell depends on a close association between two events— depolarization of the postsynaptic cell (to relieve the Mg^{2+} block) and binding of glutamate to the NMDA receptor—NMDA receptors detect coincidences. A neural mechanism that detects coincident events (associations) is an attractive model of memory because association is the essence of classical conditioning in animals and of the inference of causal relations in humans.

Experimentally, initiation of LTP can be separated from its long-term maintenance. For example, compounds that inhibit protein synthesis have no effect on the initiation of LTP in CA_1 neurons, but appear to block its maintenance. Evidence obtained by several groups has indicated that entry of Ca^{2+} through NMDA receptor channels initiates LTP in CA_1 neurons by activating protein kinases. Candidates include Ca^{2+}/calmodulin–dependent protein kinase II and protein kinase C. Pharmacological inhibitors of these protein kinases inhibit the initiation of LTP.

Distinct processes underlie the maintenance of LTP. It has been demonstrated that once LTP is initiated, persistent activation of NMDA receptors or of postsynaptic Ca^{2+}-dependent protein kinases is not required for its continued expression. Recent analyses suggest that a persistent alteration in presynaptic function—that is, a persistent increase in the amount of glutamate released on stimulation of presynaptic nerve terminals—may underlie at least part of the long-term increase in synaptic efficacy that characterizes LTP. These presynaptic changes might reflect alterations in presynaptic protein kinases, voltage-gated channels, or proteins associated with synaptic vesicle function.

How these changes in presynaptic efficacy might occur remains an open question. Because the initiation of LTP in CA_1 hippocampal neurons requires activation of postsynaptic NMDA receptors, there must be some retrograde signal to the presynaptic neuron. Current candidates for such a retrograde signal include lipophilic signaling molecules that could diffuse out of the postsynaptic neuron, for example, nitric oxide or arachidonic acid and its metabolites. This postulated requirement for a retrograde signal suggests that the postsynaptic neuron has a continuing role in the maintenance of LTP as well. The apparent dependence of LTP maintenance on new protein synthesis suggests that maintenance processes involve regulation of gene expression. The possibility that long-term changes in the presynaptic neurons are required for the maintenance of LTP suggests important analogies with invertebrate models of long-term facilitation described below.

LTP has also been described at many other synapses in the brain. Different mechanisms are involved in mediating the initiation and expression of LTP compared with those established for the CA_1 neuron of the hippocampus. For example, activation of NMDA receptors is not required for the production of LTP in CA_3 hippocampal neurons.

Long-Term Sensitization in *Aplysia*

A proposed invertebrate model of nonassociative memory involves long-term sensitization of a simple neural reflex—gill withdrawal—in the sea mollusk *Aplysia*. In brief, a noxious stimulus, such as head shock, causes sensitization of a protective gill-withdrawal reflex such that, for a period of hours after the shock, stimulation of the skin near the animal's siphon causes an exaggerated retraction of the animal's gills. Work by Kandel, Schwartz, and colleagues has indicated that cyclic AMP–dependent protein phosphorylation mediates aspects of long-term sensitization at both the cellular and behavioral levels.

According to a simplified version of this model, head shock causes an interneuron to release an unknown neurotransmitter onto the presynaptic terminal of the siphon skin sensory neuron that is a component of the gill-withdrawal reflex. In cell culture of *Aplysia* neurons, all of the effects of this transmitter are mimicked by serotonin. Within the presynaptic terminal, administration of serotonin causes the generation of cyclic AMP and the activation of cyclic AMP–dependent protein kinase. Cyclic AMP–dependent protein kinase then phosphorylates a specific type of K^+ channel (termed the *S-channel*) or a protein that regulates this channel. The S-channel is normally involved in repolarization of the neuron after an action potential. Phosphorylation renders these channels less likely to open in response to depolarization, thus strengthening and prolonging the depolarization of the presynaptic terminal. This increases the entry of Ca^{2+} into the terminal, leading to increased neurotransmitter release, and thereby increases the strength of the synaptic connection with the motor neuron, which retracts the gill.

Although relatively prolonged sensitization can be caused by a single head shock, repeated shocks or repeated administrations in culture of serotonin to the sensory neuron can cause facilitation that lasts several days. It has been proposed that such long-term facilitation depends on phosphorylation of a CREB-like protein by cyclic AMP–dependent protein kinase, which leads to expression of as yet unknown genes that act to stabilize the strengthened synaptic connection. It is striking that a single signal—activation of the cyclic AMP pathway—mediates both short-term and long-term facilitation; that is, that one intracellular pathway (which leads to activation of cyclic AMP–dependent protein kinase) bifurcates to affect short-term facilitation (via phosphorylation of ion channels and probably of other proteins such as the synapsins) and long-term facilitation (via phosphorylation of CREB-like proteins and altered gene expression within the nucleus).

Although facilitation of a simple neural reflex in a mollusk is not a complete model of memory, the mechanisms involved—a short-term change in synaptic efficacy produced by protein phosphorylation and a long-term change produced by activation of new gene expression—are likely to be similar to processes occurring in the mammalian brain.

SELECTED REFERENCES

Bekkers JM, Stevens CF: Presynaptic mechanism for long-term potentiation in the hippocampus. Nature 346:724–729, 1990

Comb M, Hyman SE, Goodman HM: Mechanisms of trans-synaptic regulation of gene expression. Trends Neurosci 10:473–478, 1987

Evans RM, Arriza JL: A molecular framework for the actions of glucocorticoid hormones in the nervous system. Neuron 2:1105–1112, 1989

Goodman RH: Regulation of neuropeptide gene expression. Annu Rev Neurosci 13:111–128, 1990

Hershey JWB: Protein phosphorylation controls translation rates. J Biol Chem 264:20823–20826, 1989

Huganir RL, Greengard P: Regulation of neurotransmitter receptor desensitization by protein phosphorylation. Neuron 5:555–567, 1990

Kacmarek LK, Levitan IB: Neuromodulation: The Biochemical Control of Neuronal Excitability. New York, Oxford University Press, 1986

Kandel ER, Schwartz JH: Molecular biology of learning: modulation of transmitter release. Science 218:433–442, 1982

Lefkowitz RJ, Hausdorff WP, Caron MG: Role of phosphorylation in desensitization of the β-adrenoceptor. Trends Pharmacol Sci 11:190–194, 1990

Madison DV, Malenka RC, Nicoll RA: Mechanisms underlying long-term potentiation of synaptic transmission. Annu Rev Neurosci 14:379–398, 1991

Malinow R, Tsien RW: Presynaptic enhancement shown by whole-cell recordings of long-term potentiation in hippocampal slices. Nature 346:177–180, 1990

Mitchell PJ, Tjian R: Transcriptional regulation in mammalian cells by sequence-specific DNA binding proteins. Science 245:371–378, 1989

Montminy MR, Gonzalez GA, Yamamoto KK: Regulation of cAMP-inducible genes by CREB. Trends Neurosci 13:184–188, 1990

Morgan JI, Curran T: Stimulus-transcription coupling in the nervous system. Annu Rev Neurosci 14:421–452, 1991

Nestler EJ, Greengard P: Protein Phosphorylation in the Nervous System. New York, Wiley, 1984

Nestler EJ, Greengard P: Protein phosphorylation and the regulation of neuronal function, in Basic Neurochemistry, 4th Edition. Edited by Siegel GJ, Agranoff B, Alber RW, et al. New York, Raven, 1989, pp 373–398

Nguyen TV, Kobierski L, Comb M, et al: The effect of depolarization on expression of the human proenkephalin gene is synergistic with cAMP and dependent upon a cAMP-inducible enhancer. J Neurosci 10:2825–2833, 1990

Sheng M, McFadden G, Greenberg ME: Membrane depolarization and calcium induce c-*fos* transcription via phosphorylation of transcription factor CREB. Neuron 4:571–582, 1990

Chapter 5

Drug-Induced

Neural Plasticity:

How Psychotropic

Drugs Work

Over the past several decades, important advances have been made toward a biological understanding of psychiatric illnesses. Many of these advances have occurred through studies of the effects of drugs on the nervous system. At a basic level, drugs are extremely useful probes of neural functioning; moreover, drugs serve as important bridges between basic research and clinical therapeutics. To date, it has been possible to identify specific neuronal populations in the brain that are involved in the actions of certain psychotropic drugs and possibly in the pathogenesis of psychiatric disorders (see Chapter 3). It has also been possible to identify specific molecular targets of drug action within these neurons.

Psychiatric research has focused particular attention on the monoamine neurotransmitter systems, in large part because antipsychotic and antidepressant drugs, psychostimulants, opiates, and hallucinogens have each been shown to directly or indirectly alter the synthesis, transport, storage, release, reuptake, or degradation of one or more of the monoamines, or to interact with one or more of the many subtypes of monoamine receptors located throughout the brain. More recently, attention has been focused on other neurotransmitter systems as

---

Text defined by vertical rules in the left margin involves advanced concepts and can be skipped by readers interested in a more general overview of the field, without loss of the overall message of the book.

well, notably acetylcholine, neuropeptides (e.g., endogenous opioid peptides), and excitatory and inhibitory amino acids. Despite these advances, however, most of the important clinical actions of psychotropic drugs cannot be fully accounted for simply on the basis of neurotransmitter and receptor regulation.

Two observations have important implications for understanding drug mechanisms: 1) Most drugs used clinically in psychiatry require chronic administration to be effective (e.g., antidepressants, antipsychotics, lithium, and atypical anxiolytics). 2) Drugs of abuse require repeated administration to produce tolerance and dependence. These observations indicate that the initial interactions of these drugs with their immediate molecular targets in the brain (e.g., of imipramine with norepinephrine and serotonin reuptake transporters or haloperidol with dopamine receptors) are not the ultimate mechanisms responsible for their important clinical effects. Rather, these clinical effects would appear to result from slow-onset adaptive changes that occur within neurons as a response to the initial interactions. We can now hypothesize, based on the information outlined in Chapter 4, that postreceptor events—namely, activation of intracellular messenger pathways and regulation of neural gene expression—play the central role in underlying long-term adaptive changes in neuronal function relevant to psychotropic drug action. In this way, the clinically important actions of psychotropic drugs can be viewed as drug-induced neural plasticity.

To test this hypothesis, it is necessary that the field of neuropsychopharmacology broaden its scope from a narrow focus on the synapse (neurotransmitters and receptors) to studies of events occurring within neurons themselves. In particular, it will be necessary to characterize the role of intracellular signal transduction mechanisms (involving, for example, G proteins, second messenger systems, protein kinases, protein phosphatases, and their numerous phosphoprotein targets such as ion channels, receptors, cytoskeletal proteins, and transcription factors) in mediating long-term changes in neuronal function produced by psychotropic drugs and to understand how these mechanisms are altered under pathological circumstances. This will not be an easy task. The intracellular pathways that underlie the chronic effects of psychotropic drugs on the nervous system are extremely complex. The multiplicity of synaptic inputs on individual neurons means that the functional activity of any given neuron in the brain depends on the activity of a large number of incoming signals. Because neurotransmission at this large number of synapses may be subserved by many different types of neurotransmitters and receptors, numerous distinct intracellular messenger pathways are likely involved in regulating that neuron's activity. These inputs must be integrated by the neuron to regulate a large number of physiological processes, including its membrane properties, its metabolic status, its responsiveness to subsequent synaptic inputs, and the number and strengths of its synaptic outputs.

It will be even more difficult to make inferences about the pathophysiology of psychiatric disorders based on drug mechanisms. The complexity of the brain's intercellular connections, with their multiplicity of interconnected control systems and feedback loops, means that therapeutically effective drugs may be acting on neurons several steps removed from any "pathophysiological lesions." For example, the dopamine antagonism of most effective antipsychotic drugs is consistent with the hypothesis that dopaminergic pathways regulate, either directly or indirectly, neurons that can produce psychotic symptoms. It cannot be concluded, however, that schizophrenia is caused by a primary problem in dopamine neurons or dopamine receptors. This concern is particularly serious for mental disorders, such as depression and schizophrenia, that are probably etiologically heterogeneous, where the fundamental pathophysiological problem may differ across patient groups with only "downstream" neuronal consequences in common.

The fact that circuits between neurons, as well as biochemical circuits within neurons, must process and integrate complex information reveals an extraordinary degree of interdependence of signaling systems at both the intercellular and intracellular levels. The implication is that a perturbation in one system will influence many others. Moreover, chronic perturbations in a system may lead to homeostatic adaptations in numerous other systems to compensate for the original perturbation. This means that a drug that produces its immediate action on a certain signal transduction pathway in a given neuronal cell type will produce short- and long-term alterations in the functional activity of many other signal transduction pathways in that neuron, as well as acute and chronic alterations in multiple signal transduction pathways in other neurons. Understanding these downstream and often temporally delayed effects of psychotropic drugs, and by analogy the effects of other environmental perturbations of the brain, is at the center of achieving a molecular understanding of psychiatry.

These points have important implications not only for the understanding of basic drug mechanisms and pathophysiology, but also for potential drug design. If, for example, we assume that all classes of antidepressant drugs (including tricyclic antidepressants, monoamine oxidase inhibitors, and atypical drugs) ultimately produce their therapeutic effects by a similar "downstream" mechanism (that this may be so is suggested by the fact that all of these drugs have similar time courses of efficacy and are effective for similar if not identical groups of patients), it follows that drugs with markedly different initial molecular targets in the brain can eventually elicit identical adaptive changes within the same populations of neurons. However, the initial molecular targets of a drug are critical determinants of its specificity and, therefore, many of its side effects. Knowledge of relevant downstream mechanisms may permit us to screen more effectively for new classes of therapeutic agents with fewer side effects or, perhaps, to design more specific drugs with more rapid time courses of action. Some of these novel drugs could conceivably exert their initial effects on the brain through interactions with intracellular messenger proteins.

Molecular approaches to psychiatry are beginning to be used by an increasing number of investigators to study the mechanisms of action of diverse types of psychotropic drugs on the brain. This chapter provides brief progress reports of current, ongoing research into four classes of drugs: antidepressants, antipsychotics, anxiolytics, and drugs of abuse. Although clearly at early stages of development, the studies illustrate the promise that this line of investigation has for the future of psychiatry.

MOLECULAR MECHANISMS UNDERLYING ANTIDEPRESSANT AND ANTIMANIC DRUG ACTION

One of the most significant advances in clinical psychiatry this century has been the introduction of antidepressant and antimanic medications. This has given us the ability to treat the majority of individuals with mood disorders. Nonetheless, additional antidepressant and antimanic drugs are needed for the sizable number of individuals who remain resistant to current treatments or who cannot tolerate their side effects. Unfortunately, several decades after their first clinical applications, the mechanisms by which antidepressant and antimanic drugs produce their therapeutic effects remain poorly understood. An improved understanding of their actions should help in the development of new drugs and may contribute to the understanding of the basic pathophysiological disturbances that cause depression and mania.

Most studies of antidepressant drugs have demonstrated that they have their most pronounced effects on monoamine neurotransmission. Early studies of antidepressant action concentrated on their immediate and direct effects on the nervous system. Imipramine and all other tricyclic antidepressants were found to inhibit the reuptake of norepinephrine and/or serotonin in varying ratios. More recently, antidepressants that specifically inhibit the reuptake of serotonin (e.g., fluoxetine) have been introduced into clinical practice. Because reuptake is the primary mechanism by which the synaptic actions of monoamines are terminated, the tricyclic antidepressants and fluoxetine-like drugs acutely increase the amount of norepinephrine and/or serotonin within synapses.

In early studies, the other major class of antidepressant drugs was also shown to affect monoamine neurotransmission. Iproniazid (no longer used clinically because of hepatotoxicity), phenelzine, and tranylcypromine were found to inhibit monoamine oxidase, an enzyme that metabolizes monoamine neurotransmitters. Because this enzyme is found in presynaptic terminals (see Chapter 3), its inhibition would prolong the life of monoamine neurotransmitters found in the presynaptic cytoplasm and thereby increase the amount of neurotransmitter available for packaging into synaptic vesicles and subsequent synaptic release.

In contrast to these antidepressants, the antihypertensive drug reserpine was shown to decrease monoaminergic transmission. Reserpine causes leakage of norepinephrine, serotonin, and dopamine out of synaptic vesicles and inhibits their reloading. The extravesicular monoamines are then metabolized by monoamine oxidase. Clinically, it had been observed that approximately 15% of patients treated chronically with reserpine developed a syndrome indistinguishable from naturally occurring depression.

Taken together, these observations led to a simple hypothesis that depression is due to inadequate monoamine neurotransmission, and that clinically effective antidepressants work by increasing the synaptic availability of monoamines by either blocking their removal from the synapse (tricyclic and related antidepressants) or inhibiting their intracellular breakdown (monoamine oxidase inhibitors). This hypothesis, advanced by Schildkraut and others, initially focused on norepinephrine, but was later extended to include serotonin as well. These early hypotheses were heuristically very important in the development of biological models in psychiatry. However, they were overly simplistic and have given way to newer hypotheses.

A major problem with all versions of these early "monoamine deficiency" hypotheses was the observation that the inhibitory actions of antidepressants on monoamine reuptake or on monoamine oxidase activity are immediate, whereas clinical efficacy requires weeks of treatment. This therapeutic delay has led more recently to the view that it is chronic adaptations in brain function, rather than increases in synaptic norepinephrine and serotonin, per se, that underlie the therapeutic effects of antidepressant drugs. The focus of research on antidepressant mechanisms has, as a result, shifted increasingly from the immediate effects of antidepressants to effects that develop more slowly. Although the focus of pharmacological research on antidepressants is shifting from acute to chronic actions, the anatomic focus has remained unchanged: monoamine projection systems are still considered to be the most important candidates for serving as the anatomical substrates of antidepressant action.

Why Are Monoamine Systems Likely to Be Critical Targets of Antidepressant Action?

Although the simple hypothesis that antidepressants work by relieving a monoamine deficiency is no longer considered adequate, the pharmacological data on which the hypothesis rested are rather compelling evidence for the importance of monoamine systems: virtually all effective antidepressant drugs have prominent interactions with the noradrenergic and serotonergic systems. Moreover, research groups continue to obtain pharmacological evidence in vivo for the importance of monoamine systems. There is, for example, recent clinical evidence that working serotonergic systems are important for the maintenance of an antidepressant response to fluoxetine, as will be discussed in greater detail later in this chapter.

At a more basic level, the various noradrenergic and serotonergic projection systems from the brain stem are organized in a way that makes them attractive candidates for being involved in the pathophysiology of depression and in the action of antidepressant drugs. Recall from Chapter 3 that these systems, although derived from a relatively small number of cell bodies, project widely to the cerebral cortex, limbic system, hypothalamus, and brain stem. Hypothesized abnormalities in such systems might explain how antidepressants relieve symptoms referable to widely divergent brain regions. Such symptoms include sleep disturbances, which might be referable to the brain stem or hypothalamus; diminished or increased appetite and diurnal variation in mood, which may be referable to different nuclei within the hypothalamus; depressed mood, which is likely to reflect abnormalities of the limbic system; altered cognition (including guilt, pessimism, and diminished self-esteem), which is likely to reflect abnormal functioning of the cerebral cortex; and psychomotor retardation or agitation, which may be explained by altered function of the basal ganglia or limbic system. Because of their wide projections, monoamine systems in the brain are unique in their ability to affect signal processing within all of these various brain regions. In addition to the norepinephrine and serotonin projections, which, based on the pharmacological data, have long been the focus of antidepressant research, the dopamine neurons projecting from the ventral tegmental area of the midbrain to the limbic forebrain are known to have powerful effects on mood and, as will be discussed later in this chapter, are likely to be the neurons on which psychostimulants act to produce euphoria. Based on what is known to date, it is not possible to state whether one or another monoamine projection system is the primary target of antidepressant action because they interact significantly with one another, such that dysfunction (or antidepressant effects) originating in one of the monoamine systems will likely be reflected in the others.

Chronic Adaptations in Monoamine Systems to Antidepressant Treatments

The chronic effects of antidepressant drugs that have been most intensively investigated are those that occur in monoamine neurons or their postsynaptic targets. Over the past 15 years, a wealth of studies have demonstrated that chronic antidepressant administration affects the turnover of monoamine neurotransmitters and regulates multiple types of monoamine receptors in the brain. These studies, largely performed in laboratory rats, have given rise to a new set of hypotheses to account for antidepressant action. All of these hypotheses correlate the delay in clinical antidepressant efficacy in humans with one or more slow-onset adaptive changes in neurotransmitter turnover or receptor sensitivity in laboratory animals.

Although many antidepressant-induced adaptive changes in monoamine neurons or their targets have been identified, none of the changes identified to date represents a convincing mechanism of antidepressant action. The first part of the discussion that follows considers some of the specific technical challenges that have made this research difficult. The second part provides an overview of the best-established long-term adaptive changes that antidepressants have been shown to induce in the brain. The discussion highlights the need for future research aimed at identifying postreceptor mechanisms by which antidepressants alter brain function.

One specific difficulty in this area of research lies in determining whether experimental findings in laboratory animals can be generalized to humans. This difficulty arises from the fact that changes in levels of most neurotransmitters, neurotransmitter receptors, or intracellular messenger systems cannot presently be measured in specific brain regions of living human patients, although advances in imaging techniques may one day enable such determinations. As a result, human studies have relied on indirect methods, such as measuring monoamine metabolite levels in cerebrospinal fluid, blood, and urine (a method with many confounding variables as well as low sensitivity and specificity) and measuring neurotransmitter receptors in peripheral blood elements such as platelets or white blood cells (which are of questionable relevance to neurons in the brain).

One method used to overcome this difficulty is the pharmacological challenge paradigm, where receptor up- or down-regulation is inferred from an increased or decreased ability of a challenge drug to induce a particular effect. For example, the neuroendocrine response to the acute administration of yohimbine (an α_2-adrenergic antagonist) has been used to estimate sensitivity of central α_2-adrenergic receptors. But even this method may not detect critical changes in the relevant neurons and, in practice, has not provided robust pathophysiological data.

An additional problem in interpreting the significance of drug-induced changes in neurotransmitter turnover and receptor sensitivity in the rat brain is the lack of adequate animal models of depression. It is quite possible that the brain of a depressed human responds differently to a drug treatment than the brain of an unaffected human or a normal rat. Indeed, administration of antidepressants to humans without depression produces no discernible effects other than the usual side effects. The difference between the brain of a normal organism and that of a depressed organism may explain, at least in part, the difficulty that investigators have had in confirming, in depressed humans by means of pharmacological challenge studies, the drug-induced changes in receptor sensitivity predicted by studies of normal rats. It therefore remains unknown whether regulation of monoamine turnover or receptors as demonstrated in rats correlates with antidepressant response in depressed patients. If neurotransmitter or receptor regulation were the actual mechanism by which antidepressants produced their therapeutic effects, one would hypothesize that among depressed patients the predicted regulation would occur in those who respond to drug treatment, but not in nonresponders. This hypothesis needs to be tested, but our ability to do so probably awaits improved imaging technologies.

Finally, most studies of antidepressant regulation of the monoamine systems to date have relied by necessity on relatively inexact measurements, even in animals. This is particularly true for studies of monoamine receptors, which have been based, almost exclusively, on ligand binding studies. Drug-induced changes in ligand binding are, by themselves, difficult to interpret; such changes could reflect altered levels of receptor synthesis, altered subcellular distribution of a constant number of receptors that changes the number of receptors available for ligand binding, or covalent modification (e.g., phosphorylation) of a constant number of receptors that changes the ability of the receptors to bind ligand. The recent cloning of multiple subtypes of these receptors, and the anticipated preparation of specific antibodies, will enable a much more complete analysis of antidepressant regulation of receptor function. Such advances will make it possible in the future to study antidepressant regulation of 1) monoamine receptors at the messenger RNA (mRNA) and protein levels, 2) receptor phosphorylation, 3) the life cycle of the receptor within subcellular compartments of the neuron, and 4) the intracellular mechanisms underlying the actions of antidepressant drugs on these receptors.

Regulation of noradrenergic systems by antidepressant drugs. Among the most consistently observed effects of chronic antidepressant administration in animals has been the down-regulation of postsynaptic β-adrenergic receptors, first reported by Sulser and colleagues in 1976 (see Figure 5–1). Virtually every class of antidepressant treatment, including chronic electroconvulsive seizures (ECS), produces this effect in cerebral cortex and other regions of the rat brain. Down-regulation of β-adrenergic receptors can be viewed as a homeostatic response to the acute actions of antidepressant drugs.

That is, by increasing synaptic levels of norepinephrine acutely, antidepressants would, over time, increase the drive on homeostatic mechanisms to decrease β-adrenergic receptor levels and thereby restore noradrenergic signal transduction within the postsynaptic neuron back toward baseline levels. (The intracellular mechanisms controlling levels of β-adrenergic receptors will be discussed later in this chapter.)

One serious problem with the "β-adrenergic receptor hypothesis" is that a number of indirect findings call into question whether down-regulation of β-adrenergic receptors, per se, exerts an antidepressant effect. A number of atypical antidepressants (e.g., bupropion) are clinically effective but do not down-regulate β-adrenergic receptors in the rat brain. Furthermore, some compounds that regulate β-adrenergic receptors do not exert the effects on clinical depression that might be predicted if β-adrenergic receptor regulation were directly relevant to mood elevation: thyroid hormone can be helpful as an adjunct therapy for depression despite the fact that it augments rather than diminishes β-adrenergic receptor function, whereas yohimbine, a compound that facilitates the development of β-adrenergic receptor down-regulation in response to tricyclic drugs, does not augment the clinical efficacy of these compounds.

Chronic treatment with some antidepressants also appears to influence α_2-adrenergic receptors in the brain, although less reproducibly than β-adrenergic receptors. Recall from Chapter 3 that α_2-adrenergic receptors largely function as autoreceptors on presynaptic noradrenergic nerve terminals; activation of these receptors by norepinephrine decreases the amount of the transmitter released in response to subsequent nerve impulses. There is some evidence, both preclinical and clinical, to suggest that chronic administration of tricyclics and certain other antidepressants leads to down-regulation of α_2-adrenergic receptors, possibly as a homeostatic response to drug-induced increases in synaptic levels of norepinephrine. Down-regulation of these receptors would reduce negative feedback by norepinephrine on presynaptic cells and could lead to an increase in overall norepinephrine release.

Antidepressant-induced down-regulation of both β- and α_2-adrenergic receptors is difficult to rationalize if these two processes are assumed to be involved in the therapeutic mechanism of drug action, because they appear to have opposing effects on noradrenergic signal transduction. In the chronic antidepressant-treated state, when both β- and α_2-adrenergic receptors are down-regulated, it is not clear whether the postsynaptic neuron is "seeing" more, less, or the same amount of norepinephrine-induced signaling than before drug administration. Similar considerations complicate interpretation of other drug-induced changes in neurotransmitter receptors, as will be seen throughout this chapter. At present, it is not known whether down-regulation of β- and α_2-

adrenergic receptors will prove to be epiphenomena or critical mechanisms of antidepressant action. Although it will not be easy to understand the implications of drug regulation of multiple receptors, it will be necessary to do so if we are to establish the mechanism of action of psychotropic drugs in the nervous system.

In addition to regulating adrenergic receptors, chronic antidepressant treatments alter the synthesis of norepinephrine in the brain. All major classes of antidepressant treatments, including chronic ECS, decrease levels of tyrosine hydroxylase in the locus coeruleus. These decreased levels would be expected to decrease the capacity of noradrenergic neurons to synthesize norepinephrine. However, the clinical relevance of this finding remains unknown; clinical studies of norepinephrine turnover have relied on measurements of norepinephrine metabolites in body fluids, a methodology that is too coarse to detect meaningful changes in particular central neurons. One possibility is that down-regulation of norepinephrine synthesis may be relevant to certain subtypes of depression in which an overactive noradrenergic system may contribute to depressive symptomatology. This, of course, remains conjectural.

Regulation of serotonergic systems by antidepressant drugs.   Chronic antidepressant treatments also produce changes in serotonergic neurotransmission within the brain. Most types of antidepressant drugs down-regulate 5-HT_2 receptors as determined by ligand binding assays, which would tend to decrease serotonergic neurotransmission. Such down-regulation of 5-HT_2 receptors can be viewed as a homeostatic response to increased synaptic levels of serotonin, similar to the mechanisms implicated for down-regulation of the adrenergic receptors. However, the relevance of 5-HT_2 receptor down-regulation to the clinical effects of antidepressants must be questioned, because chronic ECS up-regulates 5-HT_2 receptors, and some drug treatments that down-regulate 5-HT_2 receptors are not antidepressant.

Antidepressants have also been found to facilitate serotonergic synaptic transmission at certain cortical and hippocampal synapses, as determined by electrophysiological recordings. The mechanism underlying this augmentation of serotonergic neurotransmission remains unknown, but may be mediated via 5-HT_{1a} receptors. This hypothesis provides the conceptual basis for the use of newly developed 5-HT_{1a} agonists (e.g., gepirone) as antidepressants. The clinical antidepressant efficacy of such compounds must await more extensive clinical trials. As with noradrenergic systems, the complexity of changes in serotonin systems makes it difficult to determine whether chronic antidepressant treatments lead to increases, decreases, or no change in levels of overall serotonin effects on particular neurons in the brain. Moreover, as in the case of norepinephrine, the effect of serotonin on particular neurons will vary depending on the receptor types that the neuron expresses.

Clinical evidence, alluded to earlier in this chapter, provides further support for the importance of serotonergic systems in antidepressant action. In a majority of patients whose depressive episodes had been treated effectively with fluoxetine, rapid depletion of tryptophan (which impairs the activity of serotonin systems in the brain by removing the substrate for serotonin synthesis) leads to a relapse of the depression; such relapses can then be reversed with restoration of tryptophan levels. Further animal and human studies are now needed to determine 1) the precise manner in which serotonin systems exert this effect, 2) whether the therapeutic actions of other antidepressant drugs are similarly dependent on functional serotonergic systems, 3) whether other neurotransmitter systems (e.g., norepinephrine, dopamine, acetylcholine) must also be intact for maintenance of an antidepressant response, and 4) whether other therapeutic effects of fluoxetine (e.g., antipanic, antiobsessional) are similarly dependent on intact serotonin systems.

Chronic Adaptations in Intracellular Messenger
Pathways in Response to Antidepressant Treatments

The inability to account for antidepressant action solely on the basis of neurotransmitter turnover and receptor regulation raises the possibility that post-receptor events play a critical role in mediating the clinical actions of these drugs. This possibility is consistent with the view advanced earlier in this chapter and in Chapter 4 that intracellular messenger pathways and their regulation of neural gene expression play the central role in mediating long-term adaptations in neuronal function. Even the adaptations in monoamines and monoamine receptors discussed in the preceding sections, whether or not they are therapeutically relevant, are likely to be mediated via these intracellular pathways. These considerations have led an increasing number of investigators to begin to examine antidepressant-induced regulation of intracellular messengers and neuronal gene expression. The preliminary findings indicate that such studies will result in a much more complete view of the effects exerted by antidepressant drugs on brain function.

Figure 5–1 illustrates a general scheme by which antidepressants induce chronic adaptations in neuronal function. According to this scheme, antidepressants induce acute changes in the activity of specific neurotransmitter-receptor systems in the brain. The relevant acute actions of antidepressants may well involve increasing synaptic levels of the monoamine neurotransmitters (by inhibition of monoamine reuptake or degradation) as discussed previously, although additional (as yet unidentified) acute actions of these drugs cannot be excluded. Acute changes in neurotransmitter-receptor function would lead to numerous changes in the functional state of the target neurons via intracellular signal transduction pathways (see Figure 2–6). (In Figure 5–1, the cyclic AMP system is illustrated, but other intracellular signaling pathways could also be affected.) Among these changes would be relatively slowly developing alterations in gene expression, alterations that would become increasingly prominent with chronic drug administration. Such changes in gene expression would lead to long-term changes in the functional properties of the target neurons by influencing the expression of specific types of neuronal proteins. At present, the critical target proteins for antidepressant action must be considered to be unknown.

Information concerning long-term regulation of signal transduction pathways by antidepressants has been best studied for the noradrenergic system, which can serve as a model system. It must be emphasized, however, that similar types of changes would be expected for the serotonin system, as well as for many other types of neurotransmitters in the brain. Moreover, it is important to recognize that postreceptor changes that occur in response to acute effects on one neurotransmitter system within a given neuron would alter the actions on that neuron of all other neurotransmitter receptors that utilize the same intracel-

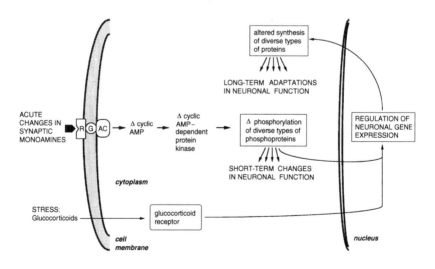

FIGURE 5–1. Schematic illustration of the postsynaptic actions of antidepressants in the brain. The figure illustrates how primary actions by antidepressant drugs at the level of the synapse could lead to multiple longer-term changes in brain function through the regulation of intracellular messenger pathways and neuronal gene expression. See text for further discussion. R = receptor. G = G protein. AC = adenylate cyclase.

lular signal transduction pathways. This is an example of heterologous regulation of receptor function (see Chapter 4).

Adaptations in the β-adrenergic signal transduction pathway. Based on studies of peripheral tissues, it has been shown that prolonged stimulation of β-adrenergic receptors leads to a cascade of changes throughout the β-adrenergic receptor signal transduction pathway, some of which are mediated at the level of gene expression. Acutely, β-adrenergic receptor activation, acting via the G protein G_s, stimulates adenylate cyclase, cyclic AMP–dependent protein kinase, and the phosphorylation of specific substrates for the protein kinase. This leads (via the phosphorylation of ion channels, metabolic enzymes, etc.) to numerous effects on target cells and also initiates a series of more subtle effects that become increasingly pronounced with continued receptor activation. For example, prolonged receptor activation leads to short-term desensitization of the β-adrenergic receptor mediated via receptor phosphorylation. Prolonged receptor activation is also known to induce the translocation of cyclic AMP–dependent protein kinase into the cell nucleus, where it appears to produce alterations in the expression of specific target genes, including those for β-adrenergic receptors and G proteins.

Increased synaptic levels of norepinephrine that occur in response to tricyclic antidepressants and monoamine oxidase inhibitors would be expected to lead to prolonged activation of β-adrenergic receptors and could conceivably initiate a similar cascade of intracellular adaptations in the brain. Indeed, some similar types of changes have been shown to occur in the brain in response to certain antidepressants. The observed down-regulation of β-adrenergic receptors could be mediated via changes in receptor expression, phosphorylation, and/or subcellular distribution, possibilities that can now be studied directly. Moreover, chronic antidepressant administration has been shown recently to alter levels of specific G protein subunits and to cause the translocation of cyclic AMP–dependent protein kinase into the nucleus in rat cerebral cortex.

Although adaptations in the β-adrenergic receptor signal transduction system are not likely to account for all aspects of antidepressant action, the mechanisms described here serve to illustrate the types of complex changes that probably contribute to the clinical efficacy of antidepressant treatments. Similar studies of other receptors and postreceptor systems are needed.

Interactions Between Antidepressant Treatments and Stress

There is growing interest in the role of stress-related mechanisms in the pathophysiology of depression. A complete discussion of the neurobiology of stress is beyond the scope of this text, but a brief overview will be presented of possible antagonistic effects of stress and antidepressants on common molecular targets.

A possible relationship between stress and depression comes from several lines of evidence. One of the most replicable biological findings in psychiatry is the observation that approximately half of patients with major depression have excess cortisol secretion and impaired feedback inhibition of the hypothalamic-pituitary-adrenal (HPA) axis, which is one of the fundamental actors in the normal stress response. It has also been shown that this hypercortisolemic state resolves after successful antidepressant treatments. In addition to the HPA axis, the noradrenergic and serotonergic systems in the brain, which are prominent targets of antidepressants (as outlined in previous sections of this chapter), are also highly regulated in response to stress. Some investigators have hypothesized that environmental factors perceived by an individual as stressful may play a role in the development of depression in some cases. Moreover, behavioral stress is used in the generation of some of the better animal models of depression, for example, learned helplessness.

One of the mechanisms by which the brain reacts to both acute and chronic stress is activation of the HPA axis. As illustrated in Figure 5–2, the HPA axis is composed of 1) hypothalamic neurons that synthesize corticotropin-releasing factor (CRF) and release it into the hypophyseal (pituitary) portal circulation; 2) corticotroph cells within the anterior pituitary that respond to CRF stimulation by secreting adrenocorticotropic hormone (ACTH); and 3) the adrenal cortex, which responds to circulating ACTH by secreting glucocorticoids. Each step in this pathway appears to be involved in mediating stress effects on the nervous system. CRF-containing neurons in the hypothalamus not only affect the pituitary, but, along with other CRF-containing neurons in the brain, affect the activity of many neuronal systems. Of particular interest, CRF activates the firing of locus coeruleus neurons.

As described in Chapter 4, glucocorticoids act by binding to their cytoplasmic receptors, which induces their translocation to the nucleus, where the receptors bind to DNA to activate or repress the expression of multiple genes. Glucocorticoids are known to influence most brain regions, but have particularly dramatic effects on limbic structures such as hippocampus and amygdala. There is also some evidence that ACTH might directly influence certain neurons in the brain. The effects that chronic stress exerts on brain function, via CRF, ACTH, and glucocorticoids, could play a role in triggering some of the pathophysiological changes in brain function related to depression and other stress-related disorders (e.g., certain anxiety disorders such as posttraumatic stress disorder).

Two findings on the mechanism of action of antidepressants suggest that the relationship between the pathophysiology of depression and the mechanism of the stress response deserves further investigation. First, it has been found that glucocorticoids and antidepressants exert reciprocal effects on several aspects of β-adrenergic receptor function and therefore cyclic AMP levels in the brain (e.g., most antidepressants down-regulate β-adrenergic receptor function, whereas glucocorticoids tend to augment receptor function in some brain regions). Second, several forms of stress have been shown to produce sustained increases in locus coeruleus neuronal firing rates and tyrosine hydroxylase expression. This effect appears to be mediated via CRF-containing neurons that

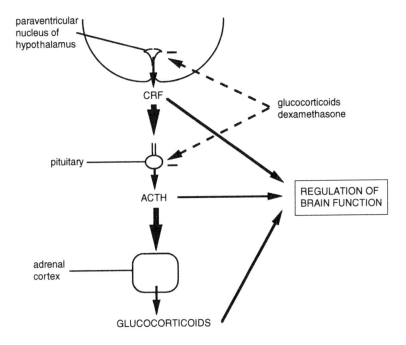

FIGURE 5–2.   Schematic illustration of the hypothalamic-pituitary-adrenal (HPA) axis. The function of the HPA axis is described in the text. Both natural and synthetic glucocorticoids (such as dexamethasone) produce negative feedback at the level of corticotropin-releasing factor (CRF) neurons in the hypothalamus and at the level of the pituitary, as shown, but also produce negative feedback on higher brain centers that regulate the HPA axis, such as the hippocampus (an important limbic structure). In about 50% of patients with major depression, the HPA axis is relatively refractory to normal feedback mechanisms. This forms the basis of the dexamethasone suppression test: high levels of glucocorticoids are released despite administration of dexamethasone. ACTH = adrenocorticotropic hormone.

project to the region of the locus coeruleus. In contrast, chronic administration of many types of antidepressants decreases the firing rate of these neurons and indeed has been shown to block the stress-induced increase in tyrosine hydroxylase expression. These findings raise the possibility that one of the clinically relevant actions of antidepressants is to reverse or prevent stress-induced increases in noradrenergic function. Similar regulation of the serotonergic system by stress and antidepressants has also been proposed. Clearly, further work is needed to study these possibilities.

Studies on the Mechanisms of Action of Lithium

Lithium is one of the most widely used psychotropic drugs, yet the mechanisms by which it exerts it antimanic and antidepressant effects after chronic administration have remained unknown. Since its introduction into clinical practice several decades ago, lithium has been shown to exert many actions on the nervous system, including acute and chronic effects on the release of serotonin and norepinephrine from nerve terminals and effects on neurotransmitter receptors and on transmembrane ion pumps. However, many of these effects occur at lithium concentrations higher than those used therapeutically. Moreover, studies at the neurotransmitter and receptor level have failed to identify the primary target of lithium action. Studies of the actions of lithium on intracellular messenger systems have been more fruitful.

Lithium regulation of the phosphatidylinositol system.   As described in Chapters 2 and 3, many neurotransmitter receptors (e.g., α_1-adrenergic, 5-HT$_2$, and muscarinic cholinergic receptors) are linked via a G protein to phospholipase C, which hydrolyzes phosphatidylinositol 4,5-bisphosphate (PIP$_2$) to yield two second messengers, diacylglycerol and inositol triphosphate (IP$_3$) (see Figure 2–9). Lithium has been shown to inhibit specific steps in the phosphatidylinositol cycle, and it has been suggested that such actions mediate lithium's antimanic and antidepressant effects. This action of lithium is shown schematically in Figure 5–3.

Phosphatidylinositol is normally synthesized from free inositol and a lipid moiety. Most cells can obtain free inositol for this synthesis directly from the plasma, but neurons cannot because inositol does not readily cross the blood-brain barrier. As a result, neurons must either recycle inositol by dephosphorylating inositol phosphates after they are generated from hydrolysis of phosphatidylinositols or synthesize it de novo from glucose-6-phosphate, a product of glycolysis. Lithium, at therapeutically used concentrations ($\sim$1 mM), inhibits several inositol phosphatases; this decreases the ability of neurons to generate free inositol either by recycling inositol phosphates or by de novo synthesis from glucose-6-phosphate. Lithium-exposed neurons, therefore, have a diminished ability to resynthesize PIP_2 after it is hydrolyzed in response to neurotransmitter receptor activation. It has been hypothesized that when firing rates of neurons are abnormally high, lithium-treated neurons will become depleted of PIP_2 more rapidly, and neurotransmission dependent on this second messenger system will be dampened. This "inositol depletion hypothesis," advanced by Berridge and others, is intriguing, because the effects of lithium might become evident only in cells with abnormally high firing rates, and because lithium would dampen the effects of multiple neurotransmitter systems and therefore could be used to treat both manic and depressive states.

However, even if this hypothesis is correct, it remains incomplete. The critical cells in the brain that are targets of lithium's therapeutic action remain unknown, and it is unclear which of the many phosphatidylinositol-dependent neurotransmitter systems must be dampened for lithium to have its therapeutic effects. Studies to date have also not adequately addressed the long-term consequences of lithium's effects on phosphatidylinositol-dependent neurotransmitter systems. Dampening of signal transduction through some or all of these systems could remain a stable feature of lithium-treated cells. Alternatively, chronic inhibition of the inositol phosphatases could lead to a buildup of active inositol phosphates, including IP_3, and thereby facilitate rather than dampen the actions of neurotransmitters on this pathway. Indeed, at present it is not at all clear whether chronic lithium administration dampens or facilitates phosphatidylinositol-dependent signal transduction in the brain.

Actions of lithium on other intracellular messenger pathways.   Chronic lithium administration also produces long-term changes in other intracellular systems in the brain. Chronic lithium administration has been shown to alter 1) the coupling of a number of neurotransmitter receptors to G proteins, 2) the expression of $G_{i\alpha}$ (and possibly other G protein subunits) and subtypes of adenylate cyclase, and 3) cyclic AMP–dependent and Ca^{2+}-dependent protein phosphorylation in specific brain regions. Each of these changes would be expected to alter the functional activity of multiple neurotransmitter signal transduction pathways in the brain, just as would be expected for lithium regulation of the phosphatidylinositol system. Studies are now needed to search for possible additional effects of chronic lithium administration and to determine which of these effects is relevant to the treatment of manic-depressive illness.

It should also be noted that lithium acutely inhibits adenylate cyclase in most tissues, including brain. Although the concentrations required to exert this effect in the brain appear to be higher than clinically relevant levels, this effect of lithium does appear to account for some of its peripheral side effects. Lithium inhibits the normal activation of adenylate cyclase by thyroid-stimulating hormone and antidiuretic hormone, which may partly explain its antithyroid effects and its tendency to cause defects in the ability to concentrate urine.

Future Directions

Given the complexity and interdependency in neurotransmitter, receptor, and intracellular messenger systems in the brain, it is likely that the antidepressant and antimanic actions of clinically useful psychotropic drugs do not lie in the modification of a single neuronal cell type or single protein but, rather, involve regulation of the expression and functional properties of multiple proteins in multiple neuronal cell types. Although such complex mechanisms of action make this a difficult area of investigation, study of intracellular messenger systems and neuronal gene expression may make it possible to gradually unravel the complex actions of antidepressants and lithium that together result in their multiple therapeutic effects on brain function.

Identification of molecular mediators of antidepressants will lead to the development of novel pharmacological agents. Sites beyond the receptor level, now known to be regulated by antidepressants, can be targeted for novel antidepressant drugs in the future; these include G proteins, enzymes that control second messenger levels (e.g., cyclic nucleotides, Ca^{2+}, and phosphatidylinositol and arachidonic acid metabolites), protein kinases and protein phosphatases, and specific phosphoproteins.

FIGURE 5–3 *(at right)*.   Effects of lithium on the phosphatidylinositol cycle. Many neurotransmitter receptors are linked via a G protein (G) (G_i, G_o, or G_q) to phospholipase C, which hydrolyzes phosphatidylinositol 4,5-bisphosphate (PIP_2) to generate two second messengers, diacylglycerol and inositol 1,4,5-triphosphate (Ins 1,4,5-P_3, most often abbreviated as IP_3). After it acts to release Ca^{2+} from intracellular stores, Ins 1,4,5-P_3 is metabolized to forms that may be inactive in neural signal transduction, including inositol 1,3,4,5-tetraphosphate (Ins 1,3,4,5-P_4). These forms are eventually metabolized to produce three different inositol monophosphates (Ins 4-P, Ins 1-P, and Ins 3-P), which differ only by the carbon atom to which the phosphate group is linked. Synthesis of inositol from glucose-6-phosphate also must pass through an inositol monophosphate intermediate.

All inositol monophosphates are metabolized by an enzyme termed *inositol monophosphate phosphatase*. This enzyme is inhibited by lithium at therapeutic concentrations. As a result, in the presence of lithium, these inositol monophosphates cannot be dephosphorylated to yield free inositol, which is required to regenerate phosphatidylinositol 4,5-bisphosphate. Also shown in the figure is the ability of lithium to inhibit an additional enzyme in this cycle (inositol polyphosphate 1-phosphatase), which is required for two metabolic steps earlier in the recycling pathway. It is important to emphasize that the functional consequences of lithium's action on the phosphatidylinositol cycle after chronic drug administration remain unknown.

Identification of molecular mediators of antidepressant action raises the possibility that abnormalities in one or more of these pathways may contribute to affective illness, at least in some patients. Finding such genetic abnormalities will lead to improved diagnostic measures that will enable affective illnesses to be subdivided into etiologically meaningful categories. Certain genetic abnormalities could then be used to predict a positive therapeutic response to a particular class of antidepressant medication. These possibilities are discussed in greater detail in Chapter 7.

MOLECULAR MECHANISMS UNDERLYING ANTIPSYCHOTIC DRUG ACTION

The introduction of antipsychotic drugs in the 1950s had a profound effect on the practice of psychiatry; however, the existing drugs are ineffective for many

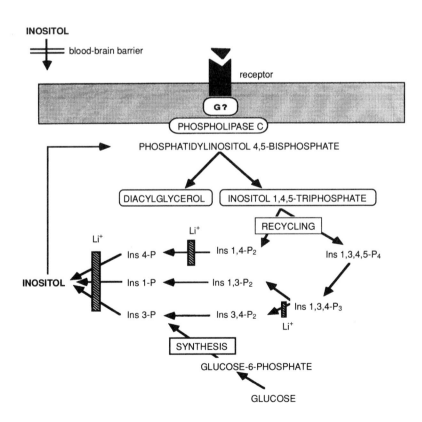

schizophrenic patients and only incompletely effective for most. These drugs also have many serious side effects, especially on extrapyramidal movement. It is a high priority, therefore, to develop better antipsychotic medications. This is an especially difficult task in that neither the mechanisms of action of antipsychotic drugs nor the pathogenesis of schizophrenia or other psychotic disorders is well understood.

Antipsychotic Drugs and Dopamine Receptors

It is clear from behavioral experiments in animals and receptor binding studies in vitro that the major shared property of all commonly used antipsychotic drugs is their action as dopamine receptor antagonists. Although antagonist drugs do not produce independent receptor-mediated effects, they can produce profound effects in vivo by interrupting ongoing dopaminergic synaptic transmission. The major dopamine receptor type that has historically been considered the target of antipsychotic drugs in the brain is the dopamine, type 2 (D_2), receptor; however, as described in Chapter 3, a recent spate of molecular cloning studies have revealed multiple new dopamine receptor types, and even more probably remain to be discovered. Thus, firm conclusions about the role of any given dopamine receptor type in antipsychotic drug action cannot yet be made.

The typical (haloperidol-like) antipsychotic drugs have equal efficacy in treating psychotic symptoms, but differ markedly in potency, as reflected by differences in the average dose of each drug needed to achieve a maximal therapeutic effect. For example, haloperidol is approximately 50 times more potent than chlorpromazine, but both drugs are equally effective if used at equipotent doses. Some of the strongest evidence purporting to show that D_2 receptor blockade is a critical contributor to the therapeutic action of the antipsychotic drugs was the observation that the antipsychotic drugs bind to the D_2 receptor with a rank order of in vitro binding affinity that roughly parallels their rank order of clinical therapeutic potency (e.g., haloperidol > perphenazine > chlorpromazine). This argument is somewhat circular, however, because in some cases clinical dosing has been based on behavioral or in vitro measurements of D_2 receptor occupancy. Nonetheless, no similar parallel was seen between clinical potency and the affinity of antipsychotic drugs for other neurotransmitter receptors (e.g., the D_1, 5-HT_2, muscarinic cholinergic, or adrenergic receptors) that were known when this type of research was done in the 1970s.

As mentioned above, however, two novel D_2-like receptors have recently been discovered by molecular cloning. These receptors are currently called the D_3 and D_4 receptors, but it is possible that a change in nomenclature will prove necessary. These new receptors are considered D_2-like because D_2, D_3, and D_4

receptors all have high affinity for similar drugs, all have a similar molecular structure, and all likely have inhibitory effects on adenylate cyclase (see Chapter 3), although this is unclear for D_3 at present. In contrast, the D_1 and newly cloned D_5 dopamine receptors roughly share a different set of drug affinities and molecular structures, and both activate adenylate cyclase.

A striking observation from the point of view of antipsychotic drug action is that the atypical antipsychotic drug clozapine is a relatively weak D_2 receptor antagonist, but has a 10-fold higher affinity for the D_4 receptor. Combined with the growing evidence that clozapine may exhibit unique clinical efficacy in schizophrenia, this observation has called into question a necessary role for D_2 receptor antagonism in antipsychotic drug action and has focused attention instead on the D_4 receptor. It must be borne in mind, however, that clozapine interacts with many other neurotransmitter receptors, including D_1 and D_3, 5-HT$_{1c}$ and 5-HT$_2$, muscarinic cholinergic, and α_1-adrenergic receptors. This makes it difficult to argue that any single effect of the drug is responsible for its clinical properties.

It is believed that the therapeutic actions of antipsychotic drugs are exerted in the mesolimbic and mesocortical dopamine projections in the brain. Recall from Chapter 3 that these systems arise from dopamine cell bodies in the ventral tegmental area and project to limbic and cerebral cortical regions (e.g., nucleus accumbens, cingulate cortex, and prefrontal association cortex). This hypothesis of antipsychotic drug action, although widely accepted, is by no means proven. It is not yet clear what function these mesolimbocortical dopamine projections subserve under normal conditions or how they might contribute to the production or attenuation of psychotic symptomatology. It is possible, for example, that these dopaminergic projections are not the ultimate targets of antipsychotic drug action, but are one or several synapses away from such neurons and are involved only indirectly.

Regardless of the dopamine or other neurotransmitter receptor(s) involved in antipsychotic drug action, a salient observation about the clinical use of all antipsychotic drugs, including clozapine, is that they achieve maximum clinical efficacy over a period of weeks. Therefore, in analogy to the antidepressant drugs and lithium, it is necessary to distinguish the acute effects of antipsychotic drugs from the effects that they exert with chronic administration. Because antipsychotic drugs inhibit neurotransmission through dopamine receptors (and other neurotransmitter receptors) immediately on entering the brain, whereas the clinical effects are considerably delayed, dopamine receptor antagonism must be conceptualized as an initial molecular interaction of antipsychotic drugs that produces as yet unknown chronic adaptations in brain function that are the actual proximate causes of therapeutic improvement.

Although blockade of dopamine receptors appears to be one mechanism by which adaptations in neural functioning that decrease psychosis can be produced, there is no reason to suspect that dopamine receptor antagonism is the unique mechanism by which such adaptations can be achieved. Drugs acting initially through other receptor types or directly on intracellular signal transduction pathways could, in principle, converge on the same mechanisms of neural adaptation. Indeed, there are currently major efforts to discover nondopaminergic antipsychotic drugs with the hope of designing drugs free of extrapyramidal side effects. One approach has been to develop drugs with multiple receptor effects, including both serotonin and dopamine receptor antagonism. Another approach involves the development of novel ligands for the sigma (σ) receptor and for the N-methyl-D-aspartate (NMDA) glutamate receptor. Recall from Chapter 3 that psychotomimetic opioids (e.g., benzomorphans) act on σ receptors and that phencyclidine (PCP) appears to exert a psychotomimetic effect by blocking the NMDA receptor channel. This raises the theoretical (and as yet untested) possibility that drugs that act as σ receptor antagonists or that modify transmission through NMDA receptors may be antipsychotic.

Receptor Actions Relevant to Side Effects of Antipsychotic Drugs

The direct actions of antipsychotic drugs on dopamine and other receptors can be related directly to a variety of their side effects. The most troubling side effects of the drugs appear to be mediated via the nigrostriatal dopamine pathway, which consists of dopamine cell bodies in the pars compacta of the substantia nigra and their projections to the caudate and putamen (striatum). The nigrostriatal pathway partly overlaps with the mesolimbocortical projection system, but provides essentially unique innervation to regions of the striatum involved in extrapyramidal motor function. Death of nigrostriatal dopamine neurons is the pathophysiological cause of Parkinson's disease. Blockade of D_1 and D_2 receptors in the striatum by typical haloperidol-like antipsychotic drugs produces extrapyramidal side effects, including dystonias and parkinsonism, and over time may produce tardive dyskinesia. These extrapyramidal side effects create major limitations on the use of standard antipsychotic drugs in clinical practice. If D_2 receptors were the critical initial target of antipsychotic drugs in the brain, it might not be possible to design antipsychotic drugs devoid of extrapyramidal effects because D_2 receptor blockade clearly adversely affects extrapyramidal motor function. However, clozapine produces antipsychotic effects without significant extrapyramidal side effects. This may reflect the fact that clozapine has a high affinity for D_4 receptors but, unlike haloperidol-like antipsychotic drugs, has a low affinity for D_2 receptors. Current evidence suggests that in contrast to D_2 receptors, which are expressed at high levels in the striatum as well as on limbic and cortical neurons, D_4 receptors are localized largely to limbic areas and have very low levels of expression in the striatum. This raises the exciting possibility that a new generation of selective D_4 receptor antagonist drugs could be designed that produce the adaptations in the brain that lead to an antipsychotic effect, but that do not cause extrapyramidal side effects. Solid information about this intriguing possibility must await the development of new selective drugs as well as the identification of additional dopamine receptor subtypes.

Tardive dyskinesia, which is presumably mediated via D_2 receptor antagonism in the nigrostriatal dopamine system, is a particularly important extrapyramidal side effect of typical antipsychotic drugs that severely limits their chronic administration. It is defined as abnormal movements (usually choreoathetoid) that occur typically after exposure to antipsychotic drugs for several months. In contrast to drug-induced parkinsonism, which is reversible on cessation of the antipsychotic drug, tardive dyskinesia persists for many months, at a minimum, after drug discontinuation and may be permanent.

Tardive dyskinesia has been explained in the past by the dopamine receptor supersensitivity (up-regulation) known to occur in the striatum in response to chronic antipsychotic drug treatment. This hypothesis is based on the idea that if blockade or failure of dopaminergic transmission (e.g., by neuroleptics or in Parkinson's disease) causes a paucity of movement, the abnormal involuntary movements of tardive dyskinesia might be explained by excess dopaminergic function. This explanation is not convincing. First, tardive dyskinesia may be evident even when patients are maintained on antipsychotic drugs and have their putatively supersensitive dopamine receptors blocked. Dopamine receptor supersensitivity is probably a more relevant explanation for the transient withdrawal dyskinesias that can occur after antipsychotic drug doses are decreased or discontinued. Second, based on postmortem receptor binding studies in patients with a history of antipsychotic drug treatment, it appears that levels of D_2 receptors return to baseline within several months after the drugs have been discontinued. Tardive dyskinesia can nonetheless continue unabated for many years in the absence of ongoing neuroleptic treatment. Two alternative hypotheses are now in the early stages of testing. One states that tardive dyskinesia is due to an alteration in intracellular signal transduction pathways within dopamine neurons that remains aberrant even after the D_2 receptors themselves have returned to normal levels. The other hypothesis states that antipsychotics produce (as yet undetected) cell death in dopamine neurons, or other neurons in the basal ganglia, by directly or indirectly generating toxic chemical species such as free radicals or by disinhibiting excitotoxic effects of glutamate receptors (see Chapter 3), which are found, in addition to dopamine receptors, on striatal neurons.

The tuberoinfundibular system is the third major dopamine system in the brain; it arises in the arcuate nucleus of the hypothalamus and projects to the pituitary gland. In this system, dopamine acts via D_2 receptors as an inhibitor of the synthesis and release of prolactin by pituitary lactotrophs. By antagonizing dopamine in this system, antipsychotic drugs produce hyperprolactinemia and galactorrhea in some patients.

Antipsychotic drugs also cause side effects by binding to various nondopaminergic neurotransmitter receptors. The low-potency antipsychotic drugs (e.g., chlorpromazine, thioridazine, mesoridazine) are strong antagonists of muscarinic cholinergic receptors and thereby produce side effects such as dry mouth and constipation. Clozapine also has substantial anticholinergic potency, but it produces excessive salivation, possibly via actions at serotonin receptors. Postural hypotension is produced by antagonism of α_1-adrenergic receptors. Antipsychotic drugs with substantial affinity for this receptor include the low-potency compounds, as well as clozapine. Sedation appears to result from antagonism of several neurotransmitter receptors, including α_1-adrenergic, muscarinic cholinergic, and histamine, type 1 (H_1), receptors. Because of substantial affinity for these receptor types, the low-potency antipsychotic drugs are quite sedating. An additional property of many antipsychotic drugs is blockade of L-type Ca^{2+} channels on neurons, cardiac muscle, and smooth muscle. Thioridazine and pimozide are particularly potent Ca^{2+} channel blockers, which may explain their cardiac toxicity (prolongation of the QTc interval with risk of torsade de pointes ventricular tachycardia). It has been hypothesized that the side effect of retrograde ejaculation caused by thioridazine is also due to its Ca^{2+} antagonist properties. Finally, some phenothiazine antipsychotic drugs are "calmodulin antagonists": they inhibit the ability of Ca^{2+}-calmodulin complexes to activate a number of enzymes, such as certain protein kinases (see Chapter 2). However, this effect occurs at such high drug concentrations that it is very unlikely to be involved in their clinical actions.

Chronic Adaptations to Antipsychotic Drugs

A major focus of current antipsychotic research is the identification of the chronic adaptations these drugs induce in the brain that underlie their antipsychotic effects and some of their long-term side effects, such as tardive dyskinesia. Two general approaches have been used: electrophysiological and molecular.

Chronic electrophysiological adaptations to antipsychotic drugs.
Acutely, antipsychotic drugs increase the firing rate of midbrain dopamine
neurons. This effect is mediated by two mechanisms. D_2 receptors are found
both postsynaptically in the terminal fields of the nigrostriatal and mesolimbocortical projections and also presynaptically as inhibitory autoreceptors
on the dopaminergic neurons themselves. Acute blockade of the D_2 receptors
by antipsychotic drugs in both locations would increase the activity of the
dopaminergic neurons. Blockade of the presynaptic D_2 receptors inhibits the
normal negative feedback of dopamine on dopaminergic neurons. Blockade
of postsynaptic D_2 receptors in the terminal fields of these neurons leads to
inhibition of polysynaptic neuronal feedback loops that also normally exert
an inhibitory influence on the dopamine neurons.

Studies by Bunney and colleagues have demonstrated that chronic administration of antipsychotic drugs produces a very different set of effects on midbrain dopamine neurons. It appears that the neurons become so activated by the
drugs that they develop something called "depolarization block" after prolonged drug exposure. Recall from Chapter 2 that the electrical excitability of
neurons depends on voltage-dependent Na^+ channels—channels that open, and
later close (or inactivate), in response to membrane depolarization. Prolonged
excitation of neurons can potentially depolarize them to the point where their
Na^+ channels become persistently inactivated; they do not open in response to
further membrane depolarization. Under such depolarization blockade, the neurons are partially depolarized but functionally inactive because they can no
longer develop action potentials in response to excitatory stimuli.

It has been suggested that depolarization block in midbrain dopamine neurons, which would produce a prolonged inhibition of dopaminergic function, is
responsible for some of the delayed actions of antipsychotic drugs—their
antipsychotic effects as well as some of their side effects. It is of interest that
virtually all antipsychotic drugs produce this type of depolarization block in
dopamine neurons of the substantia nigra and ventral tegmental area, whereas
the atypical antipsychotic drug clozapine produces this effect in the ventral tegmental area only. Depolarization block in the substantia nigra could be related
to neurological side effects, whereas in the ventral tegmental area it could be
related to the antipsychotic actions of the drugs. How depolarization block
could have an impact on psychotic symptoms, however, remains unknown.

Chronic molecular adaptations to antipsychotic drugs. An additional
approach has been to focus on the regulation of intracellular messenger
pathways and gene expression by antipsychotic drugs. For example, the
prototypical antipsychotic drug haloperidol has been shown to activate the

expression of several genes and to repress others in the striatum, limbic system, and frontal cortex. To date, all of this work has been performed in laboratory rats, making it a complex task to extrapolate the data to psychotic humans. Nonetheless, the results raise the intriguing possibility that the slow-onset therapeutic effects of antipsychotic drugs reflect changes in gene expression that alter the levels of particular proteins in specific neuronal populations in the brain (see Figure 5–4).

One change that has received considerable attention is up-regulation of dopamine receptors, particularly the D_2 receptor, in a number of brain regions. This effect was demonstrated originally by many laboratories by receptor binding studies in rats and in postmortem human brain tissue. More recent studies have shown that such up-regulation of the D_2 receptor occurs at the mRNA level. Up-regulation of the receptors can be seen as a homeostatic response to overcome dopamine receptor blockade.

The combination of numerous acute and chronic effects of antipsychotic drugs on the dopamine system highlights the current difficulty in knowing whether chronic drug administration leads to an increase, decrease, or no change in levels of overall dopaminergic neurotransmission. Consider the following information. Acutely, antipsychotic drugs would antagonize dopamine receptors. Does the receptor up-regulation seen with chronic drug use partially or completely reverse the continued drug antagonism of the receptors, or does it overshoot to lead to overall receptor supersensitivity? What is the combined effect of depolarization block and receptor supersensitivity? Moreover, changes in overall dopamine receptor function would have different effects on dopaminergic neurotransmission depending on whether these changes occur in the dopamine neurons themselves or in their target neurons. For example, overall up-regulation of dopamine receptors in dopamine cell bodies and terminals would decrease dopaminergic neurotransmission because these receptors are primarily inhibitory autoreceptors, whereas receptor up-regulation in target neurons would increase dopaminergic neurotransmission. Clearly, much additional work is needed to sort out these complex factors to determine precisely what type of change in dopamine function is associated with antipsychotic action.

In addition to regulation of the D_2 receptor, it has long been known that the gene for the endogenous opioid peptide precursor proenkephalin and the genes for other neuropeptides such as neurotensin are activated in the striatum by haloperidol. It might also be expected that antipsychotic drugs cause adaptations in the expression of many neurotransmitter receptors in addition to the D_2 receptor. These effects of antipsychotic drugs on gene expression are presumably mediated by initial inhibition of dopaminergic neurotransmission followed by consequent changes in intracellular messenger pathways in target neurons, as outlined in Chapter 4. According to this scheme, alterations in second messenger and protein kinase levels would produce altered phosphorylation of transcription factors, which would then lead to changes in the expression of specific target genes. One focus of current research, therefore, is to identify the specific transcription factors mediating the effects of antipsychotic drugs on gene expression. Haloperidol has been shown to stimulate the expression of certain transcription factor genes, such as c-*fos* and *zif*268, in the basal ganglia and

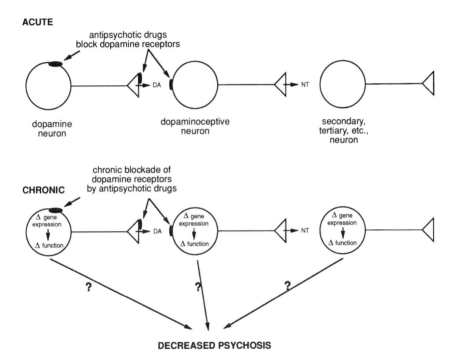

FIGURE 5–4. Schematic illustration of the possible neural targets of antipsychotic drugs responsible for their clinical actions. Typical antipsychotic drugs are thought to exert their initial effects on the brain by antagonizing dopamine (DA) receptors, present both on dopaminergic neurons themselves (cell bodies and nerve terminals) and on dopaminoceptive neurons. With prolonged exposure to the drug, it is hypothesized that persistent antagonism of dopamine receptors leads to changes in gene expression (and hence in functional properties) of the dopaminergic and dopaminoceptive neurons. Changes in gene expression and function might also occur in neurons innervated by dopaminoceptive neurons, in neurons innervated by those cells, and so on. The particular neurons in which the critical changes responsible for antipsychotic drug efficacy occur remain unknown. NT = neurotransmitter.

nucleus accumbens. Genes that may be regulated by Fos, Zif268, or other hal-operidol-regulated transcription factors might include the genes mentioned above (e.g., those for neuropeptides, receptors, G proteins, and other signal transduction proteins) or those for many other critical neuronal proteins. Some genes will be activated, and, over time, their protein products may build up to levels that are biologically significant. Other genes may be repressed, so that over time, as their mRNAs and proteins turn over, their loss may also have important biological effects.

It must be made clear that at present there is no evidence to implicate Fos, Zif268, or any other specific transcription factor in antipsychotic drug action, nor is there evidence to implicate particular target genes that might be regulated by these factors. What is critical is the idea that chronically administered antipsychotic drugs can produce marked changes in the program of gene expression of target neurons. Because of their time course, these changes are important candidates for playing a role in the therapeutic mechanism of action of antipsychotic drugs.

MOLECULAR MECHANISMS UNDERLYING ANXIOLYTIC DRUG ACTION

Anxiety is a ubiquitous symptom, and anxiety disorders represent the most common form of mental illness, with up to 15% of the population affected. The most widely prescribed and most effective anxiolytic medications are the benzodiazepines, all of which share a basic mechanism of action: facilitation of $GABA_A$ receptor function. Much of this section is therefore devoted to $GABA_A$ receptors and the mechanism of action of benzodiazepines. Attention is also given to other drugs that are used in the treatment of anxiety disorders and that influence some of the same neuronal systems.

The GABAergic System in Anxiety

Mechanism of action of benzodiazepines.   The benzodiazepines currently in clinical use all appear to act in the same way: they facilitate the actions of the inhibitory amino acid neurotransmitter γ-aminobutyric acid (GABA) by binding to $GABA_A$ receptors and inducing a conformational change that increases the affinity of the receptor for GABA. The different clinical properties of the various benzodiazepine drugs appear to depend on their relative potencies (reflected by the dose of the drug needed to achieve maximum efficacy) and their pharmacokinetics (e.g., rate of absorption, lipophilicity, route of metabolism, and elimination half-life). The heterogeneity of $GABA_A$ receptors described in Chapter 3 raises the possibility that some differences in clinical effects of various benzodiazepines might be the result of preferential binding at different $GABA_A$ receptor subtypes. However, for the currently available benzodiazepines, clinically significant receptor selectivity has not been convincingly shown. Over all, it appears likely that, at equipotent doses, all of the benzodiazepines are equally efficacious, although they may differ in side effects, with some of the higher-potency benzodiazepines, such as alprazolam, having a lower ratio of sedation to anxiolysis than the lower-potency benzodiazepines, but a greater likelihood of producing dependence.

Benzodiazepines are a major exception to the pattern established by the other psychotropic drugs discussed in this chapter. In contrast to the antidepressants, lithium, and antipsychotics, the therapeutic effects of benzodiazepines are immediate. However, their long-term actions on the nervous system are very important; they produce unwanted dependence and, in a very small minority of individuals, addiction.

A benzodiazepine receptor was first identified by radioreceptor binding assays. In analogy to older work relating antipsychotic drug effects to the D_2 receptor, there was good evidence that the high-affinity benzodiazepine receptor that was identified had relevance to clinical anxiolysis because the rank order of affinities of the benzodiazepine drugs for this receptor (e.g., clonazepam > lorazepam > diazepam > oxazepam) reproduced the rank order of clinical potencies. In other words, the relative potency of these compounds as anxiolytics could be explained by the relative avidity with which they bound to this specific receptor in the brain.

With additional investigation it was established that the benzodiazepine receptor represented a binding site on the $GABA_A$ receptor—a large multisubunit protein that serves as the main type of receptor for GABA in the central nervous system (CNS). The structure, function, and pharmacology of the $GABA_A$ receptor are described in Chapter 3. The pharmacology of $GABA_A$ receptors is complex, because several classes of psychotropic compounds bind to one of at least three distinct binding sites on the $GABA_A$ receptor complex to produce varying clinical effects (see Figure 3–3).

Benzodiazepines probably bind to a site on the α subunit of the $GABA_A$ receptor complex and thereby increase the affinity of the receptor β subunit for GABA. This facilitates the ability of GABA to activate the receptor's intrinsic Cl^- channel and consequently facilitates inhibitory neurotransmission. In the absence of GABA, benzodiazepines exert little effect on the $GABA_A$ receptor. Competitive antagonists of anxiolytic benzodiazepines have been found, such as flumazenil. These antagonists exert no independent effects on the $GABA_A$ receptor, but competitively reverse the effects of benzodiazepine "agonists" (e.g., diazepam) on receptor function. Clinically, drugs like flumazenil should prove useful in the treatment of benzodiazepine overdoses, but might be expected to precipitate withdrawal in benzodiazepine-dependent patients in analogy to the actions of opiate antagonists, such as naloxone, on opiate-dependent patients.

Another class of compounds has been identified that bind to the benzodiazepine receptor but that exert effects opposite to those of the benzodiazepines on $GABA_A$ receptor function (i.e., the drugs decrease the GABA-activated Cl^- conductance). The prototype of these drugs is β-carboline-3-carboxylate (β-CCE or β-carboline). In animal models, β-CCE is proconvulsant and proconflict. (The *conflict test* is an animal model used to screen for benzodiazepine effects. An animal presses a lever for food or water, but simultaneously receives a shock, which tends to inhibit further pressing of the lever. A state of "conflict" is said to exist between the desire for food and the expectation of punishment. Benzodiazepines are anticonflict: they release behaviors inhibited by conflict; i.e., the rat continues to eat or drink despite the threat of punishment.)

In primates, β-CCE produces dose-related increases in behavioral agitation, plasma cortisol levels, blood pressure, and heart rate. Such compounds given to human volunteers produce sympathetic arousal and intense feelings of inner tension and doom. The effects of β-CCE can be blocked by diazepam or flumazenil, suggesting that its binding site overlaps with the benzodiazepine binding site. However, β-CCE differs from pure benzodiazepine antagonists, such as flumazenil, in having physiological actions that are independent of competition with agonist benzodiazepines. These observations have given rise to a number of confusing terms for β-CCE–like compounds, such as "active antagonists" or "inverse agonists." It might be better to think of these compounds as noncompetitive antagonists of GABA, because they probably produce their physiological effects by decreasing GABA-mediated Cl^- conductance and thereby decreasing the overall amount of GABAergic-mediated inhibition in the nervous system. (By analogy, benzodiazepines would be considered noncompetitive agonists of GABA.)

Barbiturates also bind to the $GABA_A$ receptor, but at a physically separate site from benzodiazepines. Thus, both drugs can be bound to the receptor at once. Barbiturates exert an influence on receptor function similar to that of benzodiazepines: increasing the affinity of the receptor for GABA and thereby increasing the ability of GABA to activate the receptor Cl^- channel. Unlike the benzodiazepines, however, higher doses of barbiturates can directly cause opening of the Cl^- channel in the absence of GABA. This may explain why barbiturates cause more serious CNS depression (with greater likelihood of lethality) than benzodiazepines when taken in overdose. In addition to increasing the affinity of the $GABA_A$ receptor for GABA, benzodiazepines and barbiturates increase the affinity of the receptor for each other. This explains the synergy of benzodiazepines and barbiturates in causing CNS depression when they are taken together.

Hypothesized endogenous ligands for the GABA$_A$ receptor. The discovery of benzodiazepine binding sites in the brain led to the hypothesis that there might be an "endogenous diazepam" in analogy with the endogenous opioids. At present, the status of the search for an endogenous ligand remains uncertain. The first candidate compound, β-CCE, was isolated from human urine. This compound, an inverse agonist for the benzodiazepine receptor as discussed above, turned out to be a product of the extraction process rather than a true endogenous compound.

More recent candidates include a peptide, identified originally by its ability to displace diazepam from its receptor in ligand binding assays. It was, therefore, given the name *diazepam-binding inhibitor* (DBI). The peptide has since been purified from rat and human brain and subsequently cloned. When given intracerebroventricularly to rats, DBI is proconflict and its effects are antagonized by flumazenil. Structurally, however, DBI appears somewhat unusual for a putative neuropeptide. It has no clear leader sequence to enter it into a secretory pathway within neurons, and it has no dibasic residues for cleavage into smaller peptides (see Chapter 3). To date, DBI has not been accepted universally as a bona fide endogenous ligand for the benzodiazepine receptor; further research is needed.

The concept of an endogenous modulator of the benzodiazepine site is attractive in that dysregulation of such a modulator might explain certain anxiety disorders. However, it is not necessary to postulate an endogenous ligand for the benzodiazepine receptor. Unlike the opiate receptors, which turned out to be independent G protein–linked neurotransmitter receptors, the benzodiazepine binding site occurs on a molecule that is a receptor for another well-characterized neurotransmitter—GABA. In this sense, the benzodiazepine binding site could turn out to be a drug acceptor site rather than a true neurotransmitter or neuromodulator receptor. (By analogy, the serotonin transporter would be considered a specific binding site for imipramine and not an "imipramine receptor.") Moreover, if there were an endogenous benzodiazepine, why not an endogenous barbiturate as well? Whether DBI or any other molecule will prove to be an endogenous ligand for the benzodiazepine receptor remains an open question.

Effects of ethanol on the GABA$_A$ receptor. Unlike benzodiazepines and barbiturates, ethanol only produces psychotropic effects when administered in very high doses to produce high concentrations in the brain (mM versus μM or nM). Based on this observation, it has been believed that the psychotropic effects of ethanol are not related to specific receptor binding, but rather to its nonspecific effects: ethanol dissolves in cell membranes and thereby alters their fluidity. However, changes in membrane fluidity alter the ability of membrane-spanning proteins, such as receptors and ion channels, to function normally, and certain membrane-spanning proteins appear to be particularly affected by changes in their lipid milieu. Thus, many of the psychotropic effects of ethanol now appear to be mediated via selective actions on GABA$_A$ receptors.

The reasons why GABA$_A$ receptors are especially susceptible to the membrane-altering effects of ethanol are unclear. Ethanol regulates the GABA$_A$ receptor by increasing its affinity for GABA; this leads to increased GABAergic neurotransmission. Note that this action is very similar to that exerted by benzodiazepines and barbiturates, although, again, the three drugs produce this effect via distinct mechanisms. Like barbiturates, higher concentrations of ethanol can open the GABA$_A$ receptor Cl⁻ channel in the absence of GABA. Ethanol may also increase the affinity of the receptor for benzodiazepines and barbiturates, perhaps explaining the synergistic effects of these drugs on CNS depression and the clinical risk of combined exposure to the drugs. Interestingly, one recent finding raises the possibility that an individual's response to ethanol may be determined in part by the molecular characteristics of his or her GABA$_A$ receptors: two genetic strains of mice that exhibit very different sensitivities to some of the acute effects of ethanol have been shown to express forms of the GABA$_A$ receptor that display correspondingly different sensitivities to ethanol in vitro. In addition to effects on GABA$_A$ receptors, there is some evidence, although more preliminary, that ethanol may influence brain function via direct inhibitory actions on certain glutamate receptors and voltage-dependent Ca^{2+} channels.

The fact that benzodiazepines, barbiturates, and ethanol have related actions on a common receptor type (the GABA$_A$ receptor) probably explains their cross-tolerance. *Cross-tolerance* means that chronic exposure to one type of drug leads to tolerance not only to the acute effects of that drug itself, but also to other drugs as well. The term also indicates that physical dependence on one type of drug can be maintained (i.e., withdrawal can be prevented) by the other drugs. Cross-tolerance between ethanol and benzodiazepines is exploited in standard protocols for the detoxification of alcoholic persons, which generally involve "substitution" of benzodiazepines for alcohol initially (this prevents serious withdrawal syndromes), followed by a gradual tapering of benzodiazepine administration, during which time the physical dependence on the drugs slowly abates.

Tolerance to and dependence on benzodiazepines.   With chronic administration, all of the benzodiazepine drugs cause tolerance to their sedating and anticonvulsant effects, although tolerance to their anxiolytic effects does not often develop. Chronic treatment, especially with high-potency benzodiazepines, also produces dependence; discontinuation of drug treatment leads to a characteristic withdrawal syndrome, with both psychological and physical symptoms (e.g., sleeplessness, tremulousness, anxiety, paresthesias, and, in some cases, seizures).

It is important to distinguish tolerance and dependence from addiction, which is marked by inappropriate drug-seeking behaviors and compulsive nonmedical use, despite adverse consequences, as will be discussed below. Some investigators argue that although benzodiazepines commonly produce dependence, they produce addiction only rarely (and then most commonly in patients with a prior history of substance abuse). Nevertheless, concerns about benzodiazepine addiction (and confusion over tolerance versus dependence versus addiction) have led to considerable hesitance among physicians and patients alike regarding the chronic use of these effective compounds, even when indicated.

The mechanisms underlying tolerance and dependence to benzodiazepines are poorly understood. No consistent changes in the affinity or total levels of benzodiazepine or GABA binding sites have been found in the rat brain. This has led some to propose that covalent modification of the $GABA_A$ receptor, perhaps its phosphorylation, might be involved. Alternatively, tolerance and dependence may be characterized by altered expression of specific $GABA_A$ receptor subtypes with different functional properties.

Heterogeneity of $GABA_A$ receptors.   Some pharmacological actions of benzodiazepine-like compounds may be interpretable in terms of the great heterogeneity of $GABA_A$ receptors, described in Chapter 3. An inverse agonist compound designated Ro 15-4513 (but not other inverse agonists) has been found to inhibit ethanol-induced Cl^- conductance. It has also been found to reverse ethanol-induced behavioral intoxication (e.g., staggering gait and impaired righting reflex) in rats. $GABA_A$ receptors containing a certain subtype of the receptor α subunit (type 6) bind Ro 15-4513 selectively and with high affinity; this receptor subtype does not bind other benzodiazepines or inverse agonists. Strikingly, the α_6 subunit is relatively selectively expressed by cerebellar granule cells. This cerebellar localization may explain the selective antagonism of alcohol-induced motor incoordination and ataxia by this novel compound. Possible clinical utility of this compound is currently being investigated.

Given the ubiquity of the GABA system and of $GABA_A$ receptors, the remarkable specificity of benzodiazepines as anxiolytics must be explained. Clinically, anxiolysis occurs at low doses and sedation at higher doses of benzodiazepines. In animal models, anticonflict properties are evident at doses that are nonsedating. As mentioned above, patients can develop tolerance to the sedative and anticonvulsant effects of benzodiazepines without loss of anxiolytic effect. These various observations raise the question as to whether different GABA$_A$ receptor subtypes mediate the different actions of the benzodiazepines. It is also possible that the different actions of the drugs are subserved by similar receptor subtypes, but in different brain regions. An important question, then, is, Which of the many GABAergic synapses in the brain are actually relevant to benzodiazepine-mediated anxiolysis, and what are their normal functions?

Based on animal models, it has been hypothesized that the anxiolytic properties of benzodiazepines reflect their actions on neurons in the limbic system, including the hippocampus and amygdala. There are also indications that GABAergic-mediated inhibition of serotonergic and noradrenergic neurons, and their projections to the limbic system, is also involved. In contrast, it has been hypothesized that the anticonvulsant actions of benzodiazepines may be largely cortical, and their sedative actions may be mediated largely in the brain stem, although this remains uncertain.

One goal of current anxiolytic research involves the development of novel benzodiazepines with unique clinical actions. One example would be anxiolytic benzodiazepines without sedative properties; these would greatly improve anxiolytic treatment. Another example would be sedative or anticonvulsant benzodiazepines to which no tolerance develops; these could improve the treatment of sleep or seizure disorders. Finally, development of benzodiazepines to which physical dependence does not develop would reduce their major liability. Whether these various types of novel drugs are even possible remains unknown. Efforts to search for such compounds have focused on benzodiazepines specific for various GABA$_A$ receptor subtypes or on compounds with complex effects (e.g., partial agonist or mixed agonist-antagonist properties) on the GABA$_A$ receptor.

Nonbenzodiazepine Anxiolytics

Buspirone.   The azaspirodecanedione buspirone is a partial 5-HT$_{1a}$ agonist that is marketed as an anxiolytic. In animal tests, buspirone has a taming effect on rhesus monkeys, inhibits conditioned avoidance responses in rats, and reduces shock-elicited fighting in mice. It is ineffective, or at best very weak, however, as an anticonflict agent in rats and monkeys. Buspirone has not yet proven to be impressive clinically, although there are reports of its efficacy in treating generalized anxiety disorder as well as the anxiety and agitation associated with dementia. The drug seems to be ineffective in the treatment of other anxiety disorders, including panic disorder.

One feature of buspirone that distinguishes it dramatically from the benzodiazepines is that its clinical efficacy requires chronic drug exposure. It would seem, therefore, that acute actions at the 5-HT_{1a} receptor are not anxiolytic, per se, but induce long-term adaptations in brain function (e.g., altered expression of receptors or intracellular messenger proteins) that are anxiolytic.

The relatively subtle effects of buspirone on generalized anxiety and its ineffectiveness in treating other disorders raise important questions about the role of serotonergic systems in human anxiety states. Of course, major problems in studying serotonergic systems include the complexity of their pharmacology (the relatively large number of known receptor subtypes), of which much is still to be learned, and the lack of an armamentarium of selective agonists and antagonists for the different receptor subtypes. This nonetheless remains a promising area of research and drug development. It should be noted that 5-HT_{1a} agonists may prove ultimately to be more effective in the treatment of affective disorders, based on very early experience with another selective 5-HT_{1a} agonist—gepirone.

Adenosine receptor agonists. Another receptor type that may eventually prove to be a target for anxiolytic drugs is the adenosine receptor. Adenosine is a purine neurotransmitter that decreases release of many other neurotransmitters (e.g., acetylcholine, norepinephrine, glutamate, dopamine, 5-HT, and GABA) in specific brain regions through actions at its A_1 receptor. The mechanism of this inhibition is complex and includes the ability of adenosine to open K^+ channels and to inhibit the opening of Ca^{2+} channels, actions probably mediated via G proteins. The central effects of adenosine are sedative, anticonvulsant, analgesic, and anxiolytic. Methylxanthines, such as caffeine and theophylline, produce their behavioral stimulant effects largely as adenosine receptor antagonists. Caffeine is anxiogenic in normal people, but can induce frank panic attacks in patients with panic disorder. Although it is generally accepted that the actions of benzodiazepines are mediated through their binding sites on $GABA_A$ receptors, the interactions of benzodiazepines and adenosine are also a matter of interest. Adenosine and diazepam have synergistic actions, and caffeine can antagonize many of the behavioral effects of benzodiazepines. The role of adenosine in human anxiety is unclear, but adenosine receptor agonists might prove to be useful in the treatment of various types of anxiety disorders.

MOLECULAR MECHANISMS UNDERLYING DRUG ADDICTION

Drug addiction is among the most serious problems facing our society today. There are many levels of concern surrounding drug addiction, and in the last analysis they must be understood at the social and psychological levels, as well as the neurobiological level. Ultimately, of course, the psychological aspects of addiction are mediated via neurobiological mechanisms in the brain. A better understanding of these neurobiological mechanisms will provide a crucial advance in our ability to treat and prevent drug abuse and addiction. In fact, investigation of drug addiction is experimentally somewhat more straightforward than investigation of the mechanism of therapeutic action of the antidepressant, antipsychotic, and anxiolytic drugs because many key aspects of drug addiction are comparable in animals and people, whereas convincing animal models of other major psychiatric disorders are still lacking. As a result, it is more straightforward to go from molecular to electrophysiological to behavioral and eventually to clinical phenomena relevant to drugs of abuse compared with other classes of psychotropic drugs discussed in earlier sections of this chapter.

A number of concepts should be defined before turning to the neurobiology of drug addiction. *Tolerance* represents reduced drug effect with repeated administration of a drug at the same dose, or the need for an increased dose to maintain the same level of effect. Tolerance may be specific for a particular drug effect—for example, with benzodiazepines tolerance may develop to sedation but not to anxiolysis; with opiates tolerance may develop to analgesia, euphoria, and respiratory depression but not to pupillary constriction. Interestingly, with certain drugs, low levels of tolerance may occur even during exposure to a single dose; for example, during a benzodiazepine overdose, a patient may regain consciousness even while serum levels remain high enough to cause coma in naive individuals. Tolerance may be either pharmacokinetic (due to increased drug metabolism and clearance) or pharmacodynamic (due to adaptations in nervous system function, e.g., alterations in drug receptors and signal transduction pathways). For most drugs of abuse, pharmacodynamic tolerance is clinically the more important mechanism.

Another important term is drug *dependence*. In classical terms, dependence is defined as an adaptive state that develops in response to repeated drug administration and is manifested by a marked physical and/or psychological disturbance (i.e., withdrawal or abstinence syndrome) when the drug is withdrawn. The traditional distinction between physical and psychological dependence is artificial because both are mediated by neural mechanisms, possibly even similar neural mechanisms, as will be seen below.

The classical operational definitions of drug *addiction* generally required evidence of physical dependence in order to make the diagnosis. However, the requirement for physical dependence as a necessary or sufficient criterion for drug addiction must be questioned. Many drugs with no abuse potential (e.g., β-adrenergic blockers, clonidine, and tricyclic antidepressants) can produce marked physical symptoms on withdrawal. On the other hand, many people who are unquestionably severe compulsive abusers of a substance have little or no physical withdrawal syndrome on drug cessation (e.g., compulsive marijuana or cocaine users, even some alcoholic persons). A more accurate and useful approach is to define addiction as a biological, psychological, and behavioral construct at the core of which is serious compulsive use of a substance despite adverse consequences, whether or not tolerance and physical withdrawal can be demonstrated.

What we understand about these mechanisms of tolerance, dependence, and addiction is presented in this section. Opiates and cocaine are the major focus, because we know the most about the addictive mechanisms underlying these drugs.

Opiate Tolerance, Dependence, and Withdrawal

Opiates, derived originally from natural alkaloids of the opium poppy, remain one of the most widely abused substances. Acutely, they produce sedation, analgesia, and mental clouding. Although the initial response to opiates may be unpleasant (with nausea and vomiting occurring frequently), opiates produce an intense euphoria in regular users. After chronic administration, opiates elicit pronounced dependence. Use of these drugs is often compulsive, and both serious physical and mental symptoms are evident after abrupt discontinuation of chronic opiate exposure.

A major advance in our understanding of opiate addiction came in the 1970s with the discovery that the brain contains endogenous opioid peptides—the enkephalins and endorphins—that act as neurotransmitters in specific neuronal cell types, and receptors specific for these opioid peptides in target neurons (see Chapter 3). This led to the view that exogenous opiates produce their effects on brain function through interactions with the endogenous opiate receptors. As presented in Chapter 2, three major classes of opiate receptors have been identified by ligand binding studies, the μ, δ, and κ receptors, although the brain may contain additional types. These various receptor types have different regional distributions in the brain, and it has been proposed that they mediate different aspects of opiate addiction, although their precise roles under normal physiological conditions as well as in addiction remain unknown. The only way to determine the exact number of receptor types, and establish their specific anatomical and regulatory properties, will be through protein purification and/or molecular cloning, which, to date, have not succeeded in isolating opiate receptors.

A large number of regions of the CNS, rich in opiate receptors, have been implicated in acute and chronic opiate action. The dorsal root ganglion, dorsal horn of the spinal cord, periaqueductal gray, and thalamus have been implicated in the analgesic effects of the opiates. These and other brain regions, such as the locus coeruleus and amygdala, have been implicated in physical dependence on opiates and in the production of physical symptoms on opiate withdrawal.

Dopaminergic neurons in the ventral tegmental area and their target neurons, most notably in the nucleus accumbens, also rich in opiate receptors, appear to play a critical role in psychological dependence on opiates—that is, on drug reinforcement and craving. Animals will self-administer opiates directly into one or both of these brain regions, whereas lesions of these pathways block systemic self-administration of the drug. Similar results have been obtained with cocaine and other psychostimulants such as amphetamine (see below). In addition, the ability of opiates and a number of other drugs (cocaine, amphetamine, ethanol, nicotine, and Δ^9-tetrahydrocannabinol—the active ingredient in marijuana) to increase synaptic levels of dopamine in the nucleus accumbens, measured by in vivo microdialysis, correlates with their addictive potential in animals and people. These various findings have led to the view, advanced by Koob, Wise, and many others, that the ventral tegmental area and nucleus accumbens, as well as certain inputs and outputs of these neurons, are critical "brain reward regions" that mediate the positively reinforcing properties of drugs of abuse and therefore, perhaps, represent the substrate of the psychological aspects of addiction to many abused substances.

Identification of the various brain regions that are rich in opiate receptors and that are implicated in particular aspects of opiate action has led to investigations of possible biochemical changes in these regions associated with addictive phenomena. In general, these studies have been disappointing because it has not been possible to demonstrate marked changes in endogenous opioid peptides or opiate receptors that could underlie addiction. This has led to the view that adaptations in postreceptor mechanisms may play the critical role in opiate addiction, and possibly in addictive responses to other drugs as well. Indeed, increasing evidence supports a central role for adaptations in intracellular messenger pathways and gene expression in drug addiction.

Role of opiate receptors in opiate tolerance and dependence. The simplest explanation for opiate tolerance would be a decrease in the number of opiate receptors under conditions of chronic drug exposure. However, as mentioned above, it has not been possible to identify consistent changes in opiate receptor affinity or number in specific brain regions. An important limitation of all studies performed to date is that they have relied, by necessity, on ligand binding studies, which might not reveal certain types of drug-induced changes in the receptors. More sophisticated studies must await molecular analysis of the opiate receptors by cloning and biochemical approaches. Some investigators have inferred from very indirect data that chronic opiate exposure alters the phosphorylation state of the opiate receptor, which might, in turn, alter the ability of the receptor to interact with its ligands or G proteins. Although a role for opiate receptor phosphorylation must be considered hypothetical, such a mechanism would not be surprising given the evidence (discussed in Chapter 4) that phosphorylation plays an important role in mediating the functional activity of many types of neurotransmitter receptors.

Role of G proteins in opiate tolerance and dependence.   A number of laboratories have demonstrated that chronic opiate treatment alters levels of $G_{i\alpha}$ and/or $G_{o\alpha}$ in specific regions of the CNS. Because these G protein subunits are known to mediate the acute actions of opiate receptors on neuronal function, decreases in their levels would be expected to lead to functional opiate receptor desensitization (i.e., tolerance). Indeed, following chronic opiate exposure, reduced levels of $G_{i\alpha}$ have been found in the dorsal root ganglion and the nucleus accumbens.

As a seeming paradox, however, other brain regions, for example, the locus coeruleus and amygdala, show increased levels of $G_{i\alpha}$ and $G_{o\alpha}$ in response to chronic opiate exposure. Empirically, the regional differences observed in G protein regulation correlate with the effects of chronic opiate exposure on non-opiate receptor systems in these various regions (heterologous versus homologous receptor regulation). In the dorsal root ganglion, in addition to inducing desensitization to opiate agonists (i.e., tolerance), chronic opiate exposure also induces desensitization to other receptor systems that act through the same G proteins; α_2-adrenergic and serotonergic agonists also have diminished effects. Such heterologous desensitization could be accounted for by the reduced levels of $G_{i\alpha}$ and $G_{o\alpha}$ induced in the dorsal root ganglion by chronic opiate exposure. In contrast, opiates induce homologous desensitization in the locus coeruleus, a region in which chronic opiate exposure increases levels of G proteins. Further work is needed to test the validity of this hypothesis.

Role of the cyclic AMP pathway in opiate tolerance and dependence.
Early studies by Sharma, Klee, and Nirenberg in cultured cells derived from

fusions of neuroblastoma with glioma cells first implicated the cyclic AMP system in mechanisms of opiate tolerance, dependence, and withdrawal. More recent studies by Aghajanian and Nestler and their colleagues have provided direct evidence that adaptations in the cyclic AMP system represent one mechanism by which opiates induce dependence in several of their target neurons. This will be illustrated by consideration of the locus coeruleus, which has served as a very useful model to study the molecular mechanisms of opiate addiction.

Acutely, opiates inhibit the firing rates of rat locus coeruleus neurons. Tolerance develops to this acute inhibition, as locus coeruleus firing rates return toward control levels with continued opiate administration. Locus coeruleus neurons also develop dependence on opiates after chronic drug exposure, because administration of opiate receptor antagonists to opiate-dependent rats results in dramatically increased locus coeruleus firing rates in vivo. Considerable evidence now indicates that these changes in the electrical excitability of locus coeruleus neurons contribute prominently to opiate physical dependence and withdrawal in several animal species, including humans. This knowledge of opiate action in the locus coeruleus led to the introduction of clonidine, an α_2-adrenergic receptor agonist, as an effective treatment of opiate abstinence now used widely in clinical settings.

The mechanisms underlying the acute inhibition of locus coeruleus neurons by opiates have been studied with electrophysiological and biochemical techniques and are shown schematically in Figure 5–5 *(top)*. Opiates acutely inhibit locus coeruleus neurons by regulating two types of ion channels: activation of a K^+ channel and inhibition of a slowly depolarizing nonspecific cation channel. Opiate regulation of both channels is mediated through the G proteins G_i and/or G_o. Opiate regulation of the cation channel is mediated through a G protein–induced decrease in neuronal levels of cyclic AMP. Presumably, opiate-induced decreases in cyclic AMP, and consequently in cyclic AMP–dependent protein phosphorylation, lead either directly or indirectly to changes in the conductance of the slowly depolarizing cation channel. Such regulation of protein phosphorylation probably also mediates many additional effects of opiates on locus coeruleus neurons, including even some of the initial steps underlying longer-term changes associated with dependence.

In contrast to acute opiate action, chronic opiate administration up-regulates the cyclic AMP system in the locus coeruleus at each major step between receptor and physiological response (Figure 5–5, *bottom*). Chronic opiate administration has been shown to increase levels of adenylate cyclase, cyclic AMP–dependent protein kinase, and a number of phosphoproteins, including tyrosine hydroxylase, in the locus coeruleus.

The up-regulation of the cyclic AMP system in the locus coeruleus in response to chronic opiate administration can be viewed as a homeostatic control mechanism by which locus coeruleus neurons overcome persistent opiate inhibition of the cells. According to this view, the concurrent presence of morphine and the up-regulated cyclic AMP system in opiate-dependent animals would result in locus coeruleus firing rates close to control levels (i.e., tolerance). When the morphine is withdrawn abruptly (e.g., by administration of an opiate receptor antagonist), the up-regulated cyclic AMP system, unopposed by morphine, would increase the activity of locus coeruleus neurons and produce a number of symptoms of the opiate abstinence syndrome.

This scheme is supported by several lines of evidence. First, neurotransmitters that act through cyclic AMP and cyclic AMP–dependent protein kinase are known to excite locus coeruleus neurons. Second, locus coeruleus neurons from opiate-dependent animals exhibit increased intrinsic excitability and increased responsiveness to drugs that act through the cyclic AMP pathway, presumably due to the up-regulated cyclic AMP system in these cells. Third, the time course by which components of the cyclic AMP system recover during opiate withdrawal closely parallels the time courses by which withdrawal activation of locus coeruleus neurons and behavioral measures of withdrawal return to baseline during early stages of opiate abstinence. Fourth, systemic administration of agents that inhibit phosphodiesterase (this enzyme degrades cyclic AMP so that inhibitors increase cyclic AMP levels) produces a morphine-withdrawal–like syndrome in normal rats and potentiates the signs and symptoms of opiate abstinence in opiate-dependent rats. It is possible that these effects of phosphodiesterase inhibitors are mediated in part at the level of the locus coeruleus.

The opiate-induced up-regulation of the cyclic AMP system in the locus coeruleus appears to be mediated largely at the level of gene expression: opiate-induced alterations in this system (where it is possible to study them), have been shown to involve increased levels of mRNA and protein. A major focus of current research is to identify the precise molecular pathways by which opiates regulate gene expression in the locus coeruleus and thereby induce tolerance and dependence in these neurons. The transcription factor c-Fos or related proteins are possible molecular mediators of opiate action. Acutely, opiates produce a rapid decrease in levels of c-*fos* mRNA in the locus coeruleus, a decrease that persists during chronic opiate exposure, whereas precipitation of opiate withdrawal leads to a rapid increase in locus coeruleus c-*fos* expression. Similar changes in levels of the c-Jun transcription factor occur in this brain region. Regulation of the state of phosphorylation of cyclic AMP response element binding (CREB) protein—another transcription factor (see Chapter 4)—by acutely and chronically administered opiates, and during opiate withdrawal, has also been demonstrated recently. Future studies will be aimed at identifying the role played by these and other transcription factors in mediating the effects of opiates on known target proteins (e.g., G proteins, adenylate cyclase, cyclic AMP–dependent protein kinase) in locus coeruleus neurons.

More recent studies indicate that up-regulation of the cyclic AMP system may play a similar role in mediating opiate tolerance, dependence, and withdrawal in a number of other regions of the CNS, including the dorsal root ganglion, nucleus accumbens, amygdala, and thalamus. An important implication of these studies is that similar biochemical mechanisms would underlie both the physical and psychological aspects of drug addiction. According to this view, up-regulation of the cyclic AMP system (and alterations in levels of G proteins as mentioned earlier) represents a common response of a number of neuronal cell types to chronic opiate administration, with such adaptations in intracellular pathways leading to physical or psychological symptoms of addiction, or both, depending on the particular neurons involved. This further emphasizes the blurred and arbitrary distinction between physical and psychological dependence, as discussed earlier in this chapter.

Role of glutamatergic neurotransmission in opiate tolerance and dependence. The preceding discussion of opiate addiction focused on factors that are *intrinsic* to locus coeruleus neurons (i.e., up-regulation of the cyclic AMP

FIGURE 5–5 *(at right).* **Schematic illustration of the mechanisms of acute and chronic opiate action in the locus coeruleus (LC).** *Top panel:* Opiates acutely inhibit locus coeruleus neurons by increasing the conductance of a K^+ channel *(stippled)* via coupling with G_o and/or G_i, and by decreasing the conductance of a nonspecific cation channel *(hatched)* via coupling with G_i and the consequent inhibition of the cyclic AMP pathway *(downward bold arrows)* and reduced phosphorylation of the channel or a closely associated protein. Inhibition of the cyclic AMP pathway, via decreased phosphorylation of numerous other proteins, would affect many processes in the neuron; in addition to reducing firing rates, for example, it would initiate alterations in gene expression via regulation of transcription factors.

Bottom panel: Chronic administration of opiates leads to a compensatory up-regulation of the cyclic AMP pathway *(upward bold arrows),* which contributes to opiate dependence in the neurons by increasing their intrinsic excitability via increased activation of the nonspecific cation channel. In addition, up-regulation of the cyclic AMP pathway presumably would be associated with persistent changes in transcription factors that maintain the chronic morphine-treated state. Chronic opiate administration also leads to a relative decrease in the degree of activation of the K^+ channel due to tolerance, the mechanism of which is unknown. Also shown in the figure is the vasoactive intestinal polypeptide receptor (VIP-R). VIP is a major activator of the cyclic AMP pathway in the locus coeruleus.

Source. Reprinted from Nestler EJ: "Molecular Mechanisms of Drug Addiction." *Journal of Neuroscience* 12:2439–2450, 1992. Used with permission.

pathway). However, *extrinsic* factors are responsible for about half of the elevation in locus coeruleus neuronal firing rates seen during opiate withdrawal. Lesions of the nucleus paragigantocellularis, a region in the medulla that provides a major glutamatergic input to the locus coeruleus, attenuate by about 50% the several-fold increase in locus coeruleus neuronal firing rates on withdrawal in vivo. Intracerebroventricular or local locus coeruleus administration of glutamate receptor antagonists produces a similar effect.

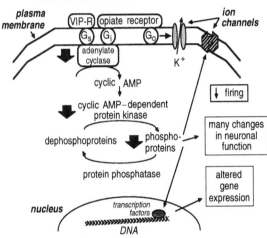

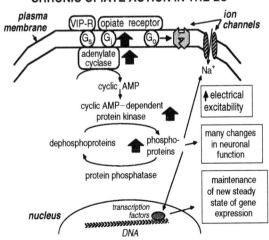

Where do the changes occur that underlie the role of the nucleus paragigantocellularis in withdrawal activation of locus coeruleus neurons, and what is their nature? These changes might occur within the locus coeruleus in nerve terminals of axons projected from the nucleus paragigantocellularis, in cell bodies within the nucleus paragigantocellularis, or in any afferents that innervate the nucleus paragigantocellularis. Indeed, chronic opiate administration up-regulates the cyclic AMP pathway in dorsal root ganglion–dorsal horn of the spinal cord (which provides a major afferent to the nucleus paragigantocellularis) and in the nucleus paragigantocellularis itself. These findings indicate that an up-regulated cyclic AMP system may contribute to opiate dependence in several neuronal cell types (as mentioned above), which summate to lead to the greatly increased firing rates of locus coeruleus neurons in vivo.

The findings also demonstrate the likely complexity of the types of mechanisms underlying opiate addiction even for such a homogeneous and "simple" brain region as the locus coeruleus, and the critical importance of considering neural networks when attempting to understand drug addiction. This view is supported further by growing evidence for a role of glutamatergic neurotransmission in opiate tolerance, dependence, and withdrawal. For example, systemic administration of glutamate receptor antagonists has been shown to attenuate the development of tolerance to and physical dependence on opiates in laboratory animals. It must be borne in mind, of course, that glutamatergic neurotransmission occurs at a large fraction of all synapses in the brain, such that these observations may indicate the requirement for multiple, intact neural networks in the development and expression of opiate addiction and not a specific role for glutamate in these phenomena.

Cocaine Addiction

Cocaine, derived as a natural alkaloid from the coca plant, acts as a psychostimulant. Like amphetamine, cocaine increases locomotor activity, increases the subjective sense of energy, and induces an intense euphoria. In higher doses, cocaine, like amphetamine, can produce psychotic symptoms including paranoid delusions. One of the most important clinical properties of cocaine is that it is intensely reinforcing; it appears to be one of the most powerfully addicting drugs known. In controlled studies, it has been shown that craving for cocaine increases dramatically with chronic use of the drug. The intensity of cocaine craving is illustrated by the fact that those addicted to cocaine are often willing to violate virtually every social taboo to obtain the drug. Animals show similar degrees of cocaine craving: given free access to cocaine after chronic exposure, some animals show little ability to moderate their cocaine use and will prefer cocaine to normal cycles of eating, drinking, and sleeping.

In contrast to withdrawal from opiates and CNS depressants, in which there may be striking derangements of many physiological parameters, most of the manifestations of cocaine abstinence in dependent individuals are subjective or manifested behaviorally. Cocaine abstinence is characterized by a protracted state of withdrawal (lasting months to years) in which intense cocaine craving (which can be exacerbated by conditioned cues), anhedonia, and high risk of relapse into active cocaine abuse are prominent symptoms. There remains, however, considerable controversy as to the precise symptoms and course of cocaine withdrawal. In past years, the lack of change in heart rate, blood pressure, or the like during cocaine abstinence had led to a mistaken idea that cocaine does not produce "physiological" dependence. In fact, as stated earlier, behavioral and psychological symptomatology reflect long-term changes in neural functioning just as physical symptomatology does.

Tolerance has been reported to develop to some of the acute actions of cocaine after chronic exposure to the drug, for example, its euphoriant and cardiovascular actions. However, the effects of chronic cocaine administration are more complicated. In contrast to many other drugs that produce only tolerance (or tachyphylaxis—a pharmacological term meaning tolerance), repeated administration of cocaine produces certain behavioral effects to a progressively greater extent in response to the same dose of the drug. This phenomenon has been referred to as *behavioral sensitization*. The locomotor-activating effects of cocaine are among the best characterized behaviors that exhibit such sensitization. Increasing evidence cited earlier also suggests that the reinforcing actions of cocaine exhibit sensitization—that is, cocaine craving increases with chronic cocaine use.

The acute action of cocaine that has received most attention is its ability to bind with high affinity to the dopamine transporter protein and to thereby inhibit the reuptake of dopamine by dopaminergic nerve terminals (see Figure 3–6). Cocaine inhibition of dopamine reuptake would be expected to increase synaptic levels of dopamine, an action confirmed in recent years by direct measurement of extracellular dopamine levels by in vivo voltammetry and microdialysis. It is generally thought, as discussed earlier, that such actions of cocaine in the ventral tegmental area–nucleus accumbens pathway mediate the reinforcing aspects of this drug. Amphetamine and methamphetamine also increase synaptic levels of dopamine, although by a different mechanism: these drugs increase the release of dopamine from dopaminergic nerve terminals.

Cocaine has other acute actions on the brain as well. It is a potent inhibitor of serotonin and norepinephrine reuptake, and these actions may play a critical role in the addictive properties of cocaine. In fact, these other actions might explain why more specific inhibitors of dopamine reuptake (e.g., mazindol, nomifensine) have not proven to be particularly reinforcing. Cocaine is also a local anesthetic, although this action is not thought to play a prominent role in its reinforcing properties.

Despite the evidence that some of the acute and chronic actions of cocaine are mediated by the ventral tegmental area–nucleus accumbens pathway, the changes that cocaine induces in these brain reward regions that underlie the long-term aspects of cocaine abuse (i.e., psychological dependence and craving) are less well established. Recently, electrophysiological alterations induced by chronic cocaine use have been demonstrated in ventral tegmental area and nucleus accumbens neurons. Chronic cocaine use renders ventral tegmental area neurons subsensitive to D_2 receptor activation, whereas it renders nucleus accumbens neurons supersensitive to D_1 receptor activation. It has been proposed that this disequilibrium in the physiological sensitivity to dopamine contributes to chronic effects of cocaine on this neural pathway. However, these changes in physiological sensitivity to dopamine occur in the absence of consistent changes in the dopamine receptors themselves (as measured by ligand binding), raising the possibility that postreceptor mechanisms may be involved.

Role of G proteins and the cyclic AMP system in psychological dependence on cocaine. Preliminary studies indicate that decreased levels of $G_{i\alpha}$ and $G_{o\alpha}$ and an up-regulated cyclic AMP system may contribute to cocaine addiction in the ventral tegmental area and nucleus accumbens. Chronic treatment of rats with cocaine results in decreased levels of these G protein subunits in the ventral tegmental area and nucleus accumbens, plus increased levels of adenylate cyclase and cyclic AMP–dependent protein kinase activities in the nucleus accumbens only. Because D_2 receptors act through G_i and/or G_o, a decrease in these proteins could account for the subsensitivity to D_2 receptor activation observed in ventral tegmental area neurons in response to chronic cocaine administration. Similarly, because D_1 receptors act through G_s and activation of the cyclic AMP pathway, increased levels of adenylate cyclase and cyclic AMP–dependent protein kinase, with a decrease in G_i/G_o, could account for the supersensitivity to D_1 receptors observed in nucleus accumbens neurons in response to chronic cocaine administration.

Common mechanisms underlying psychological dependence on opiates and cocaine. Chronic treatment of rats with morphine or cocaine produces some similar biochemical alterations in the ventral tegmental area and nucleus accumbens. These common biochemical adaptations are consistent with the increasing behavioral evidence that certain aspects of opiate and psychostimulant action exhibit "cross-sensitization": chronic treatment with one drug sensitizes the animal to certain effects of the other. Thus, as stated above, chronic morphine administration decreases levels of G_i and increases levels of adenylate cyclase and cyclic AMP–dependent protein kinase in the nucleus accumbens, as does chronic cocaine administration. In contrast, drugs without reinforcing properties have no effect on these intracellular messengers. Chronic cocaine administration and chronic morphine administration also regulate the same subset of phosphoproteins, among which are tyrosine hydroxylase and several neurofilament proteins, specifically in the mesolimbic dopamine system. Interestingly, some of these phosphoproteins show different inherent levels in inbred rat strains (Lewis and Fischer 344 rats) that exhibit different levels of cocaine, morphine, and alcohol self-administration. These various data are consistent with the possibility that these intracellular pathways not only mediate some common actions of opiates and cocaine on brain function, but also may contribute to individual genetic vulnerability to drug addiction.

Future Directions

These studies, although still at early stages, support the view that through the study of drug regulation of intracellular messenger systems and neuronal gene expression, it will be possible to learn a great deal about the precise molecular mediators of drug addiction. These studies will have a number of important implications. It should be possible to develop pharmacological agents that prevent or reverse the actions of the drugs on specific target neurons. These agents could be used to treat not only physical abstinence syndromes, but also the craving for abused substances that lies at the heart of drug abuse. Pharmacological attenuation of drug craving would represent a revolutionary step in our battle against drug addiction, which until now has relied on psychosocial treatments that are notoriously ineffective.

There are well-established differences among individuals in their risk for drug addiction. This is true for laboratory animals as well as for people. It is now feasible to begin to study the genetic basis of such individual differences by determining whether variant genetic forms of any of the identified molecular mediators of opiate and cocaine action contribute to such differences in drug preference. This approach has already yielded some success in the early studies of inbred rat strains discussed above. Identification of some of the genetic factors that predispose individuals to drug abuse would greatly advance our understanding of drug addiction, as well as eventually improve its treatment and prevention.

SELECTED REFERENCES

Aghajanian GK: Tolerance of locus coeruleus neurons to morphine and suppression of withdrawal response by clonidine. Nature 276:186–188, 1978

Avissar S, Schreiber G, Danon A, et al: Lithium inhibits adrenergic and cholinergic increases in GTP binding in rat cortex. Nature 331:440–442, 1988

Baraban JM, Worley PF, Snyder SH, et al: Second messenger systems and psychoactive drug action: focus on the phosphoinositide system and lithium. Am J Psychiatry 146:1251–1260, 1989

Berridge MJ, Downes CP, Hanley MR: Neural and developmental actions of lithium: a unifying hypothesis. Cell 59:411–419, 1989

Braestrup C, Nielsen M, Olsen CE: Urinary and brain β-carboline-3-carboxylates as potent inhibitors of brain benzodiazepine receptors. Proc Natl Acad Sci U S A 77:2288–2292, 1980

Bunney BS, Sesack SR, Silva NL: Midbrain dopaminergic systems: neurophysiology and electrophysiological pharmacology, in Psychopharmacology: The Third Generation of Progress. Edited by Meltzer HY. New York, Raven, 1987, pp 81–94

Chappell PB, Smith MA, Kilts CD, et al: Alterations in corticotropin-releasing factor-like immunoreactivity in discrete rat brain regions after acute and chronic stress. J Neurosci 6:2908–2914, 1986

Colin SF, Chang HC, Mollner S, et al: Chronic lithium regulates the expression of adenylate cyclase and G_i-protein α subunit in rat cerebral cortex. Proc Natl Acad Sci U S A 88:10634–10637, 1991

Delgado PL, Charney DS, Price LH, et al: Serotonin function and the mechanism of action of antidepressant action: reversal of antidepressant induced remission by rapid depletion of plasma tryptophan. Arch Gen Psychiatry 47:411–418, 1990

DeMontigny C: Electroconvulsive shock treatments enhance responsiveness of forebrain neurons to serotonin. J Pharmacol Exp Ther 228:230–234, 1984

Duman RS, Strada SJ, Enna SJ: Glucocorticoid administration increases receptor-mediated and forskolin-stimulated cyclic AMP accumulation in rat brain cerebral cortical slices. Brain Res 477:166–171, 1989

Gold PW, Goodwin FK, Chrousos GP: Clinical and biochemical manifestations of depression. N Engl J Med 319:348–353, 413–420, 1988

Harrelson AL, McEwen BS: Hypophysectomy increases vasoactive intestinal peptide-stimulated cyclic AMP generation in the hippocampus of the rat. J Neurosci 7:2807–2810, 1987

Heninger GR, Charney DS: Mechanism of action of antidepressant treatments: implications for the etiology and treatment of depressive disorders, in Psychopharmacology: The Third Generation of Progress. Edited by Meltzer HY. New York, Raven, 1987, pp 535–544

Henry DJ, Greene MA, White FJ: Electrophysiological effects of cocaine in the mesoaccumbens dopamine system: repeated administration. J Pharmacol Exp Ther 251:833–839, 1989

Insel TR, Ninan PT, Aloi J, et al: A benzodiazepine receptor-mediated model of anxiety: studies in nonhuman primates and clinical implications. Arch Gen Psychiatry 41:741–750, 1984

Kitayama I, Janson AM, Cintra A, et al: Effects of chronic imipramine treatment on glucocorticoid receptor immunoreactivity in various regions of the rat brain. J Neural Transm 73:191–203, 1988

Koob FF, Bloom FE: Cellular and molecular mechanisms of drug dependence. Science 242:715–723, 1988

Luddens H, Pritchett DB, Kohler M, et al: Cerebellar GABA$_A$ receptor selective for a behavioral alcohol antagonist. Nature 346:648–651, 1990

Nestler EJ: Molecular mechanisms of drug addiction. J Neurosci 12:2439–2450, 1992

Nestler EJ, McMahon A, Sabban EL, et al: Chronic antidepressant administration decreases the expression of tyrosine hydroxylase in the rat locus coeruleus. Proc Natl Acad Sci U S A 87:7522–7526, 1990

Newman ME, Lerer B: Post-receptor-mediated increases in adenylate cyclase activity after chronic antidepressant treatment: relationship to receptor desensitization. Eur J Pharmacol 162:345–352, 1989

Pritchett DB, Sontheimer H, Shivers B, et al: Importance of a novel GABA$_A$ receptor subunit for benzodiazepine pharmacology. Nature (London) 338:582–585, 1989

Rasmussen K, Beitner DB, Krystal JH, et al: Opiate withdrawal and the rat locus coeruleus: behavioral, electrophysiological, and biochemical correlates. J Neurosci 10:2308–2317, 1990

Redmond DE Jr, Krystal JH: Multiple mechanisms of withdrawal from opioid drugs. Annu Rev Neurosci 7:443–478, 1984

Schildkraut J: The catecholamine hypothesis of affective disorders: a review of supporting evidence. Am J Psychiatry 122:509–522, 1965

Sulser F: New perspectives on the molecular pharmacology of affective disorders. Eur Arch Psychiatry Neurol Sci 238:231–239, 1989

Wise RA: The role of reward pathways in the development of drug dependence. Pharmacol Ther 35:227–263, 1987

Chapter 6

Overview of

Psychiatric Genetics

The methods of recombinant DNA technology have provided tools of unprecedented power to map the loci of inherited diseases and to investigate their fundamental pathophysiology. By combining classical and molecular genetics, investigators have identified and cloned the genes responsible for an increasing number of important inherited disorders, including numerous inborn errors of metabolism, Duchenne muscular dystrophy, cystic fibrosis, and certain forms of diabetes mellitus. Moreover, investigators are now close to identifying the genes responsible for Huntington's disease, familial Alzheimer's disease, and certain forms of cancer.

By identifying and cloning the aberrant genes, it has become possible to study the defective proteins responsible for the disorders. Such advances in molecular medicine have begun to revolutionize diagnosis and should eventually have a profound impact on the treatment and even prevention of serious diseases in humans.

Vulnerability to many of the most severe psychiatric disorders appears to be heritable, and identification of the specific genes and proteins involved would similarly revolutionize the practice of psychiatry. However, despite great effort, at the time of this writing, it has not yet been possible to identify the specific genes responsible for mental disorders.

Several major factors make psychiatric genetics extremely challenging. In contrast to many nonpsychiatric disorders (e.g., cystic fibrosis, Huntington's disease, and diabetes), it is difficult to make psychiatric diagnoses with cer-

---

Text defined by vertical rules in the left margin involves advanced concepts and can be skipped by readers interested in a more general overview of the field, without loss of the overall message of the book.

tainty. This is because most psychiatric disorders are symptom complexes for which definitive diagnostic criteria are unavailable. As a result, affected and nonaffected individuals can be easily misclassified in family and genetic studies. Accurate classification is complicated by a variety of possibilities. A single genetic defect may produce markedly different phenotypes depending on interactions with other genes and environmental factors (variable expressivity). Thus, it is possible that a single gene conferring vulnerability to bipolar disorder may produce unipolar illness in one member of a family and bipolar illness in another.

Other problematic factors include the possibility that the disease gene is present, but not expressed (reduced penetrance), and the fact that some psychiatric disorders can occur at any point in an individual's lifetime, which makes it difficult to classify an individual as "unaffected" when at some future point he or she could develop the disease in question. Although models of genetic transmission can take these factors into account, these factors increase the difficulty of the analysis markedly.

Even if patients can be accurately classified phenotypically, additional difficulties remain. Many, if not all, psychiatric disorders (including major depression and schizophrenia) may well prove to be etiologically heterogeneous. This means that patients with the same illness clinically may actually have different illnesses etiologically. This situation could arise if two or more different genetic defects produce a similar phenotype. The situation could also arise if an environmentally caused behavioral abnormality clinically mimics a genetic disorder. An example of such an abnormality, which would be termed a *phenocopy,* is the surreptitious use of cocaine that mimics the highs and lows of bipolar disorder via a process unrelated to the genes that contribute to bipolar disorder.

The problem of heterogeneity is exacerbated by the relatively high frequency with which individuals with psychiatric disorders pair and have children *(assortative mating).* When assortative mating occurs, transmission of the disorder within the pedigree is bilineal, increasing the likelihood of etiological heterogeneity within the pedigree and thereby confounding the analysis.

A final and very serious difficulty is that the mode of inheritance of major psychiatric disorders may prove to be extremely complex in that classical Mendelian patterns of inheritance are generally not apparent in families with these disorders. As will be discussed later in this chapter, Mendelian traits are traits inherited as a *single major genetic locus.* As traits or disease vulnerabilities are based on increasing numbers of genes, the mode of genetic transmission becomes increasingly difficult to analyze. The purpose of this chapter is to provide a basic overview of classical and molecular approaches by which the genetic factors involved in psychiatric disorders can be studied.

CLASSICAL GENETICS

Modes of Inheritance

Normal humans possess 46 chromosomes: two copies of each of 22 different autosomal chromosomes (one copy of each inherited from the mother and the father) and 2 sex chromosomes. Females have 2 X chromosomes and males have 1 X and 1 Y chromosome. Each chromosome contains thousands of genes as well as much DNA without apparent function (see Chapter 1).

In his pioneering genetic studies, Gregor Mendel described the inheritance of certain traits of pea plants (such as green versus yellow or smooth versus wrinkled peas). In modern terms, the traits that he focused on were each inherited as a single major genetic locus. A locus is any chromosomal location of interest, ranging from a single base pair to a gene cluster. Many of the loci of interest in genetic studies are single functional genes (as they were in Mendel's studies), but they may also be fragile sites within chromosomes or DNA markers with a known location on a particular chromosome. Within the human population, there is DNA sequence variation at each genetic locus. Each possible variant is called an *allele*. The multiplicity of alleles at many genetic loci is the basis of the genetic diversity of the species.

Important human disorders inherited in Mendelian fashion (i.e., as a single major locus) include Huntington's disease, cystic fibrosis, and Duchenne muscular dystrophy. For each of these cases, the disorder appears to be caused by the inheritance of a gene with an abnormal DNA sequence or deletion of a DNA sequence at a single location in the genome.

At least in principle, the analysis of disorders related to a single major locus is relatively straightforward. However, the inheritance of many important human traits and disorders is more complex, resulting from the interaction of multiple genes. When traits result from the interaction of a relatively small number of genes, they are referred to as *oligogenic*. Disorders thought to be oligogenic include forms of essential hypertension and forms of non-insulin-dependent diabetes mellitus. A model in which a very large number of genes (technically an infinite number) contribute equally to the production of a trait is called a *polygenic* model. Truly polygenic traits are unlikely to be found in real biological systems. However, as the number of genes contributing significantly to a trait increases, the genetic analysis becomes more difficult.

Dominant, recessive, and sex-linked traits.   When a trait is inherited as a single major locus, its mode of transmission can be further analyzed. A dominant gene is an allele that can produce a phenotype when present even as a single copy—that is, a dominant allele determines the phenotype despite the presence of a second allele inherited from the other parent. This means that individuals with a dominant allele will exhibit the relevant phenotype in cases where the allele is present in either two copies (*homozygous*) or only one copy (*heterozygous*). In one classic example, brown eyes is a dominant trait, because a single copy of the brown eye allele usually leads to production of enough pigment to make the eyes brown regardless of what eye color is coded on the other allele. Among the disorders mentioned above, Huntington's disease is transmitted in dominant fashion.

A recessive allele only determines the phenotype when it is present in two copies (i.e., when the individual is homozygous for that allele). Thus, in contrast to brown eyes, blue eyes is a recessive trait, because an individual will only have blue eyes if he or she is homozygous for alleles that produce less pigment. Among the disorders mentioned above, cystic fibrosis is transmitted as a recessive disorder, requiring inheritance of two defective alleles, one from each parent.

The Y chromosome contains fewer genes than the X chromosome. When a trait or disorder involves genes present on that region of the X chromosome that has no homologous region on the Y, a special case arises: in males, but not in females, a single allele on the X chromosome will act as if it were dominant (and determine the phenotype) because males have only one allele at that locus. Females may be able to compensate because they could have a second "good" allele on their other X chromosome. Traits and disorders inherited in this fashion are referred to as *sex linked*. Sex-linked disorders such as hemophilia and the most common types of color blindness are generally seen only in males, whereas females typically act as phenotypically silent carriers of the defective allele.

The difference between dominance and recessiveness in genetic disorders has pathophysiological significance. If a genetic disorder is recessive, then two abnormal alleles are necessary for the disorder to be expressed. Pathophysiologically, the requirement for two abnormal alleles generally signifies a disorder based on loss of function. Typical recessive disorders include "inborn errors of metabolism," such as Tay-Sachs disease. Children with Tay-Sachs disease have two defective alleles of the hexosaminidase A gene and therefore lack active enzyme altogether.

In contrast, disorders transmitted as autosomal dominant traits are caused by a single defective allele despite the presence of a second normal allele. Although in some cases two normal alleles are needed to produce enough of some gene product, generally the pathophysiological significance of dominance is a "gain of function"—some gene product is being expressed in the wrong place, at the wrong time, or in destructive excess, or a gene product with a novel deleterious activity is produced. Huntington's disease is transmitted as an autosomal dominant trait; the leading pathophysiological hypothesis is that a mutant allele of a gene residing on chromosome 4 results in overproduction of a substance (perhaps an excitotoxin) that destroys specific populations of vulnerable neurons over time.

Penetrance and expressivity.   *Penetrance* refers to the probability that an individual carrying a certain gene will express the phenotype potentially conferred by that gene. If the presence of a given gene invariably produces a particular phenotype, the penetrance of the gene is said to be 100%. This is the case for Huntington's disease: carriers of the Huntington's disease gene are certain to develop the disorder if they live long enough.

For many genes, however, penetrance is less than 100%; it can be affected by the remainder of the individual's genetic background and by environmental history. For example, a second gene or set of genes might be necessary to express the disease gene. Similarly, an individual's environment can influence the expression of specific genes. One example is phenylketonuria, the clinical features of which are due to an inborn error of metabolism. As long as an individual avoids phenylalanine, the features of the disease will not develop. Hypothetical ways in which environmental factors could reduce or increase penetrance of genes for mental disorders are discussed further in Chapter 7.

PSYCHIATRIC GENETICS

Familial Transmission of Psychiatric Disorders

Despite the difficulties enumerated at the beginning of the chapter, there is strong evidence that vulnerability to many major psychiatric disorders is inherited. It has long been recognized that major psychiatric disorders aggregate in families. This has been well established by studies comparing rates of an illness in relatives of ill probands (i.e., the ill member who brought the family under study) with rates in relatives of unaffected individuals. For example, the prevalence of mood disorders in first-degree relatives of depressed individuals is at least twice that in relatives of randomly selected individuals. Bipolar disorder is even more strongly familial, with an 8%–25% incidence of the disorder in the first-degree relatives of bipolar probands, compared to an incidence of 0.5%–1% in the general population. Recent research has also demonstrated the familial nature of many other psychiatric disorders, including panic disorder, some forms of alcoholism and other types of substance abuse, schizophrenia, obsessive-compulsive disorder, and Tourette syndrome. Preliminary investigations also suggest that antisocial and borderline personality disorders also exhibit familial aggregation.

Inheritance of Psychiatric Disorders: Twin and Adoption Studies

Once it has been established that a disorder aggregates in families, further investigation is needed to determine whether the similarity among family members is explained by shared genes, shared environment (e.g., diet, socioeconomic status, education), or both. For several psychiatric disorders this issue has been addressed by twin and adoption studies. Comparison of monozygotic (identical) twins (who have 100% of their DNA in common) with dizygotic (fraternal) twins (who are genetically no more similar than any pair of siblings with an average of 50% of their DNA in common) can provide evidence for heritability; if concordance for the disorder is higher among monozygotic than dizygotic twins, a genetic contribution is likely.

Of course, studying twins raised together cannot control for the contribution of a shared environment. This has been addressed by studying the transmission of psychiatric disorders in pedigrees in which the children were adopted away early in life. In adoption studies, concordance for a disorder between the adopted child and the biological parents, rather than the adoptive parents, provides evidence of a role for heredity in the disorder. The best possible design is to study monozygotic twins reared apart by different adoptive families, but such twin pairs are relatively rare. In addition, even for twins reared apart, certain environmental factors cannot be excluded, such as factors that might have affected the twins in utero (e.g., exposure to environmental toxins, drugs, or viruses) or soon after birth. Despite their limitations, over the years, various types of adoption studies have provided strong support for the involvement of genetic factors in affective, anxiety, psychotic, and substance abuse disorders.

The use of twin and adoption studies in assessing the heritability of psychiatric illness can be illustrated by investigations of mood disorders. Twin studies of mood disorders support a strong role for heredity, which is more pronounced in bipolar disorder than in unipolar depression. Thus, for bipolar disorder, the concordance rate for monozygotic twins is 70%–85%, whereas that for dizygotic twins is about 20%. This gives a monozygotic-to-dizygotic ratio of 3.5:1. (This ratio illustrates the complexity of psychiatric genetics, as classical Mendelian inheritance would dictate a ratio of 2:1 for a dominant disease.) In contrast, for unipolar depression, the concordance rate for monozygotic twins is about 50%, whereas that for dizygotic twins is about 25%, giving a monozygotic-to-dizygotic ratio of approximately 2:1.

Mode of Transmission of Psychiatric Disorders

Once family, adoption, and twin studies demonstrate a probable genetic contribution to the pathogenesis of a psychiatric disorder, it must then be asked, What specific genetic trait(s) is being transmitted and by what mechanism? The available data indicate that for most psychiatric disorders the best model for what is inherited is a vulnerability to these disorders, not the certainty of becoming ill, nor even the exact clinical form that the illness will take.

Hypotheses about the mode by which vulnerability is transmitted can be generated using the results of *segregation analysis*. In segregation analysis, the pattern of transmission (segregation) of a trait (or disorder) is studied in extended family pedigrees, focusing on appearance of the trait both within and between generations. Ideally, analysis of the pattern of transmission can yield a model indicating, for example, whether a disorder is inherited as a single major locus or oligogenically, what the penetrance is, and, if a single major locus is involved, whether it is inherited in dominant, recessive, or sex-linked fashion. In practice, however, because of the difficulties in classifying patients as affected or unaffected and because of the potentially complex patterns of inheritance of psychiatric disorders, segregation analyses have often proven uninformative in psychiatric genetics. In many studies, it makes more sense to proceed directly to linkage analysis (discussed later in this chapter), which can be conceptualized as a special type of segregation analysis.

Where they have been performed, segregation analyses of psychiatric disorders have often revealed considerable complexity concerning the modes of transmission involved. Even where segregation analysis within one extended pedigree has produced a consistent mode of transmission for a particular psychiatric disorder, comparison of segregation analyses of the disorder derived from multiple pedigrees indicates no consistent mode of transmission (e.g., single locus versus oligogenic; dominant versus recessive versus sex linked) among the different families. This is illustrated best by consideration of bipolar disorder. Genetic vulnerability to the illness appears to be inherited as an autosomal dominant, single genetic locus in the Old Order Amish, but as a sex-linked, single genetic locus in some Israeli pedigrees. These contradictory findings are consistent with either etiological heterogeneity of bipolar disorder or errors in diagnosis.

Other psychiatric disorders have also been examined by segregation analysis. There is some evidence that Tourette syndrome may be an autosomal dominant disorder and that the gene(s) involved may also contribute to the appearance of obsessive-compulsive disorder in the same families. Preliminary evidence suggests that panic disorder is autosomal dominant in some families. In contrast, it has not been possible to arrive at a convincing model for the mode of transmission of schizophrenia. It is possible that vulnerability to schizophrenia depends on many interacting genes and that there is a strong environmental effect on penetrance. It also appears likely that, like mood disorders, schizophrenia is etiologically heterogeneous, perhaps even including nongenetic cases.

The likelihood of etiological heterogeneity of mental disorders raises several interesting considerations. One is the possibility that unrelated mutations affecting different neuronal cell types can lead to related disease phenotypes. An illustrative example from endocrinology is diabetes mellitus, where the clinical feature of glucose intolerance is due in some families to autoimmune destruction of the pancreas following viral infection and in other families to decreased responsiveness to the physiological actions of insulin in target tissues. (Of course, the clinical phenotypes of these different types of diabetes also have many distinguishing features.) Another possibility is that mutations have occurred in different genes residing on different chromosomes, but that the genes are functionally linked; for example, their protein products represent successive steps in an enzymatic pathway or different parts of a single cellular structure.

Speculation from a genetic point of view on the pathophysiology of psychiatric disorders remains premature. Considerable attention has been given to the possibility that multiple genes contribute to the development of particular mental illnesses. However, it remains possible that vulnerability to certain disorders, such as bipolar disorder, at least in some families, arises from an abnormality in a single gene, and that gene, perhaps acting in a dominant fashion, produces all of the symptoms of the disorder. Such genes might be expected to code for proteins that directly or indirectly influence a large number of functions in the brain.

The relatively high frequency of mental disorders in the general population suggests that the alleles that put an individual at risk for psychiatric illnesses may be quite prevalent in the population at large. This raises the interesting question as to why genes that lead to debilitating illnesses are so common. One possibility is that the genes confer some selective advantage to the individual under certain conditions. For example, one can imagine how a gene might alter the functional activity of a class of neurons in the brain in such a way as to lead to measured increases in energy and creativity. This would be a highly advantageous trait and one selected for strongly during evolution. However, in combination with certain genetic backgrounds and under some environmental conditions, the expression of that gene, and consequently the activity of that neuronal population, might be exaggerated to the point where mania develops. As another example, it is nearly certain that the genes that put an individual at risk for alcoholism evolved long before mankind's knowledge of fermentation. Although the normal functions of such "alcoholism-vulnerability" genes are unknown, it is conceivable that they confer a selective advantage to individuals expressing them in certain circumstances, but confer vulnerability to a deleterious phenotype (i.e., alcoholism) in other circumstances.

Just as it is now certain that genetic factors contribute strongly to the etiology of most psychiatric disorders, it is equally clear that diverse types of environmental factors also influence expression of the disorders. This is demonstrated by the finding that significant percentages of monozygotic twins (who share all of their genes) are discordant for specific illnesses. The importance of gene-environment interactions is underscored by studies of normal personality development among monozygotic twins raised apart. Genes and environment both appear to contribute to the development of many important personality traits. The identification of relevant environmental factors both for the development of mental disorders and for personality development has remained elusive, at least partly because of the increasing realization that even among siblings raised in the same family the salient environmental factors may be unshared—that is, each child in a family probably experiences the environment differently. The study of unshared environmental factors will prove extremely challenging. Eventually, however, both genetic and environmental factors and their interactions will have to be understood to have a clear picture of both normal psychological development and the pathogenesis of psychiatric disorders.

The importance of gene-environment interactions is underscored by the fact that a major area of current scientific investigation is to better understand the precise molecular mechanisms by which environmental factors of diverse types (e.g., drugs, viruses, learned behaviors) influence neuronal gene expression. This will be discussed again in Chapter 7. However, this kind of analysis can be truly successful only if it is possible to identify the genes conferring vulnerability to psychiatric disorders.

LINKAGE ANALYSIS

Although twin and adoption studies can provide strong evidence that inheritance plays a role in the development of certain psychiatric disorders, definitive evidence that vulnerability to a disorder is genetic comes from demonstrating linkage of the disease phenotype to a known genetic marker (i.e., a specific site on a chromosome) and, ultimately, from identifying the specific gene involved.

To understand linkage, it is necessary to return briefly to a review of basic genetics. In his investigations of inheritance in pea plants, Gregor Mendel found that all of the traits that he studied were inherited independently of each other and formulated the concept of "independent assortment" of traits. At the physical level, Mendel's view implied that genes are physically unrelated to each other and that germ cells could receive a random assortment of maternal and paternal genes.

In fact, Mendel chose the traits he worked on very carefully, because genes are not actually free to segregate independently. As described in Chapter 1, genes are physically connected to each other on chromosomes, which are very long molecules of DNA, each containing several thousand genes. Therefore, genes located on the same chromosome are physically linked and are a priori more likely to be inherited together. It turns out that each of the traits Mendel chose to study is on a different chromosome of the pea plant. In fact, the principle of independent assortment is more relevant to the segregation of chromosomes at meiosis than to the segregation of individual genes and therefore of individual traits. There is, however, a complicating factor: genetic recombination.

Meiosis is the process by which DNA is replicated and then apportioned to sperm and egg during the process of gamete formation. During meiosis, homologous pairs of chromosomes (i.e., the paternal and maternal copies of each chromosome) exchange DNA sequences (Figure 6–1). This process is called *genetic recombination,* or *crossing over,* and serves to increase genetic variation in the offspring. Such increased variation can be viewed as an important substrate for natural selection and evolution. On average, approximately three separate exchanges occur per chromosome during meiosis.

The probability that two genetic loci originally found on a single paternal or maternal chromosome will be separated from each other by recombination is inversely proportional to their distance from each other on the chromosome. Therefore, the closer two genetic loci are to each other (for example, the closer a disease gene is to some genetic marker), the less likely they are to be separated from each other by a recombinational event during meiosis, and the more likely they are to cosegregate with each other in the next generation. In other words, when a trait is linked to a marker, the two travel together with a frequency that is greater than expected if Mendelian independent assortment of genes (i.e., random assortment) had occurred. (In Figure 6–1, the expected cosegregation of alleles A and B on one chromosome is disrupted by recombination.)

Linkage analysis investigates whether, within a particular pedigree, a trait or disorder of interest cosegregates in significant fashion with a known genetic marker. A genetic marker is a detectable phenotypic trait or DNA sequence, which has been mapped to a known physical location on a particular chromosome. To be useful, genetic markers must be polymorphic—that is, there must be different alleles producing detectable phenotypes that can therefore be used to mark particular chromosomes and follow their segregation within a pedigree. Traditional genetic linkage markers have been traits such as ABO blood group or human leukocyte antigen (HLA) types and common disorders, such as color blindness, that have multiple detectable phenotypes and known chromosomal locations.

The demonstration of linkage to a genetic marker is strong proof that there is a genetic contribution to the trait in question. Indeed, the demonstration of linkage also identifies the approximate physical location of the locus of interest in the genome: it must be near the linked marker on the same chromosome. The closer the locus of interest is to a marker, the less frequently it will be separated from the marker by recombination and, conversely, the more frequently it will

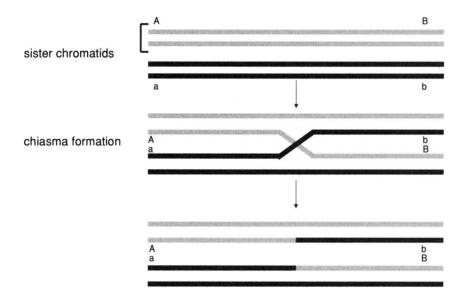

FIGURE 6–1.   Schematic illustration of genetic recombination. *Meiosis* is the process of nuclear division that leads to formation of gametes (sperm or eggs). During meiosis, cells that have the normal *diploid* number of chromosomes (i.e., two copies of each individual chromosome, one each derived from the individual's father and mother) give rise to sperm or eggs with a *haploid* number of chromosomes (i.e., a single copy of each chromosome). During meiosis, *homologous* chromosomes (the paternal and maternal copies of each chromosome) pair side by side in a zipper-like fashion. Each chromosome then replicates, giving rise to cells with four copies of each chromosome. Each of the duplicated paternal and maternal chromosomes are called *sister chromatids (top panel).*

Next, the pairing between *homologues* becomes less tight, and as they move apart, cross-shaped structures *(chiasmata)* become visible. These chiasmata, or *crossovers,* are sites at which there is a precise breakage and reunion of DNA occurring between two homologous, but nonsister chromatids *(middle panel).*

The result is an exchange of material between paternally and maternally derived chromosomes *(bottom panel).* In the example shown here, alleles A and B are originally found together on a single (paternal) chromosome, and alleles a and b are originally found together on the homologous (maternal) chromosome. Recombination produces chromosomes carrying A together with b and B together with a. Following this stage there are two successive cell divisions to yield haploid gametes. Each gamete receives an entire complement of 23 chromosomes, but the particular copy of each chromosome is determined randomly. In other words, each chromosome segregates independently.

travel together with the marker within the pedigree. It should be clear that as the number of genes that make significant contributions to a trait or disorder increases, linkage analysis becomes more difficult.

The relative likelihood that apparent linkage within a pedigree represents true linkage rather than a chance result is most often expressed as a *lod score,* where *lod* stands for logarithm of the odds for linkage. Simply put, the lod score is based on a ratio of the likelihoods for or against linkage given certain assumptions (such as degree of penetrance and whether a trait is dominant or recessive). A lod score of 3 represents odds of 1000 to 1 (where $3 = \log_{10} [1000]$) that linkage is not due to chance alone and has conventionally been accepted as statistical evidence for the linkage between two loci. However, given the way linkage studies are often performed in psychiatry, the requirement of a lod score of 3 may be too low, because multiple different phenotypic classifications are often tested for linkage, increasing the prior odds of finding linkage.

Linkage analysis is feasible only if there are an adequate number of polymorphic genetic markers spaced evenly enough throughout the genome so that all possible loci of medical interest will be linked to some marker. From this point of view, traditional phenotypic genetic markers are inadequate. Using all of the known phenotypic genetic markers, such as ABO blood groups or HLA types, a coarse linkage map covering only about 20% of the human genome can be constructed. In recent years, however, recombinant DNA technology has made it possible to generate a very large number of novel markers. This has made it possible to construct a complete linkage map of the human genome, which is continually being improved in both resolution and range with the addition of ever more molecular markers.

DNA Polymorphisms as Linkage Markers

Most modern linkage analyses do not utilize traditional phenotypic markers, but instead use DNA polymorphisms. *Polymorphic DNA linkage markers* are detectable regions of chromosomes that contain variations in primary DNA sequence (polymorphisms) within the human population. By making these differences in primary DNA sequence "visible," recombinant DNA technology has availed modern genetics of a very large number of informative markers to be used in linkage analysis.

Three of the major types of DNA polymorphisms in common use are *restriction fragment length polymorphisms* (RFLPs), *variable number of tandem repeats* (VNTRs), and a special case of the latter—*variable number of dinucleotide repeats.* RFLPs represent small regions of DNA containing sequence variations that are detectable because, as will be discussed later in this chapter, certain sequences are substrates for analytic enzymes and other sequences are not. VNTRs are regions of DNA that are composed of repetitive DNA sequences (tandem repeats) of no known function. VNTRs are useful polymorphic markers because 1) they are scattered at fairly high density throughout the genome and 2) the number of tandem repeats at any particular chromosomal location may vary within the human population, resulting in repeats that vary in length (which can be readily measured). Dinucleotide repeats are simply variable numbers of strings of the nucleotides C and A found throughout the human genome, the length of which can also readily be measured. Such markers can be used in linkage analysis by observing cosegregation of a trait of interest within a pedigree with a particular RFLP, VNTR, or dinucleotide repeat. RFLPs were the first important method of discovering DNA polymorphisms for linkage analysis and will be described in greater detail later in this section. Additional methods of identifying DNA sequence variations are also in use in genetic analyses.

Recall from Chapter 1 that genes are linear regions of DNA composed of regulatory sequences that determine where and when the gene will be expressed and coding regions (exons) interspersed with noncoding regions (introns). Genes are separated by intragenic DNA of no known function. The human genome contains approximately 3 billion base pairs of DNA. There are approximately 100,000 genes, of which perhaps 30,000 are expressed primarily in the brain. Genes range in size from 1,000 to about 200,000 base pairs and average about 10,000 base pairs. Based on these approximations, it is thought that about 10%–30% of the genome actually carries genes. Within the regulatory regions and exons of genes, the DNA sequences at homologous loci are very similar from one person to the next, although there is some sequence variation; distinct alleles of a gene reside in this type of variation. In contrast, introns and extragenic regions display considerable sequence variation, with certain of these regions being so different among individuals as to be called *hypervariable regions*. Presumably the high degree of variability in these regions suggests that they are nonfunctional: there was no evolutionary selection pressure to maintain a particular sequence. Because a high degree of polymorphism is a requirement for a useful linkage marker, hypervariable regions of the genome have been used extensively in generating DNA probes for linkage analysis.

In the RFLP method, demonstration of sequence variation among individuals depends on a class of bacterial enzymes termed *restriction endonucleases,* or *restriction enzymes.* These enzymes recognize particular sequences in DNA and cut the DNA within or near that sequence. For example, the bacterium *Escherichia coli (E. coli)* produces an enzyme called Eco R1, which recognizes the six-base nucleotide sequence GAATTC and cuts the DNA between the G and the first A on both strands (Figure 6–2). There are now scores of restriction enzymes available commercially, which recognize and cut DNA at distinct sequences. Restriction enzymes appear to have evolved to allow bacteria to cut up the DNA of invading bacteriophage viruses.

If sequence variation within the human genome occurs within the recognition sequence of a restriction enzyme, altering even a single base, the enzyme will no longer cut in that location. Alternatively, variation may create a recognition sequence where one did not exist previously. A loss or gain in a restriction site will lead to different-sized fragments when the DNA is digested by the enzyme. It is these different-sized fragments that are called RFLPs.

Figure 6–3 illustrates how individual RFLPs are identified experimentally. First, a restriction enzyme is used to digest an individual's DNA, which is typically obtained from peripheral white blood cells. Because restriction enzymes have small (several-base) recognition sequences, they may cut total human genomic DNA over a million times and produce an initially uninterpretable number of DNA fragments of widely varying sizes.

Second, the DNA fragments are ordered by size using gel electrophoresis. In electrophoresis, DNA, which is negatively charged, migrates toward a cathode in an applied electric field. Because the DNA is run through a gel that retards DNA movement, the smallest fragments of DNA migrate most quickly.

Third, specific DNA fragments are identified by Southern blotting. In this procedure, all DNA within the gel is denatured (i.e., the two complementary strands of the double helix are separated—a process termed *melting*). These now-single strands of DNA are transferred by capillary action to a membrane filter, to which they adhere irreversibly.

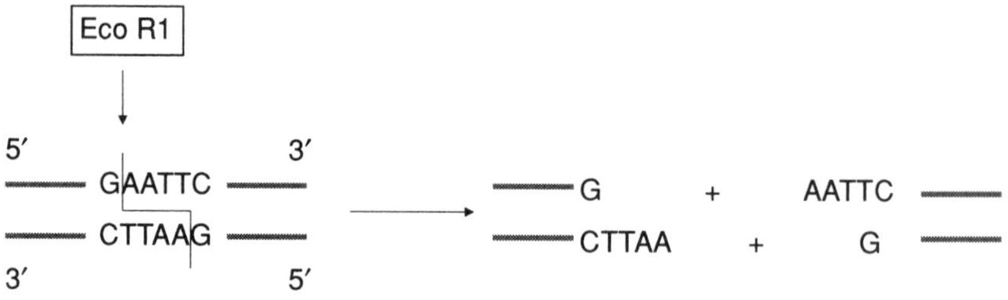

FIGURE 6–2. **Recognition sequence of the restriction endonuclease Eco R1 is shown within double-stranded DNA.** As is typical of recognition sequences for restriction enzymes, the sequence is a palindrome—that is, it is the same on both complementary strands of DNA reading from 5′ to 3′. Most restriction endonucleases have four or six base recognition sequences; a few have eight base recognition sequences. Eco R1 cuts its recognition sequence in the staggered way shown.

1. Digestion of total DNA with restriction enzymes

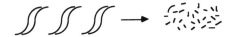

2. Separation of DNA fragments by gel electrophoresis

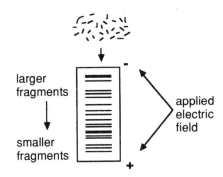

larger
fragments

smaller
fragments

applied
electric
field

3. Southern blotting

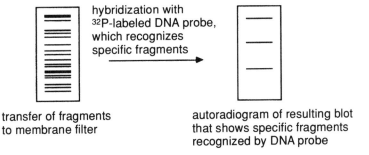

hybridization with
^{32}P-labeled DNA probe,
which recognizes
specific fragments

transfer of fragments
to membrane filter

autoradiogram of resulting blot
that shows specific fragments
recognized by DNA probe

FIGURE 6–3. Schematic illustration of experimental procedures used to identify specific DNA fragments that are recognized by a radioactively labeled DNA probe. 1) Total human DNA is digested with a restriction enzyme that cuts the DNA specifically into millions of small fragments. 2) The small fragments are separated on the basis of size by gel electrophoresis. 3) The fragments in resulting gels are transferred to membrane filters, and the filters are incubated (hybridized) with a radioactively labeled DNA probe that recognizes a specific genetic locus. The filters are washed such that radioactivity remains bound to the filters only where fragments that recognize the probe occur. The position of such radioactivity is identified by exposing the filters to X-ray film, a process termed *autoradiography.*

The filters are then incubated with a single-stranded radioactively labeled DNA probe (Figure 6–3). Recall the principles of complementary base pairing from Chapter 1. If the conditions are right, the radioactive probe will hybridize only to those DNA strands on the filter that contain sequences complementary to the probe; this will allow a double helix to form, but one of the strands will be detectable because it is radioactively labeled. These blots are then exposed to X-ray film, which reveals the location of the radioactively labeled DNA fragments. Gain or loss of a restriction site will change the migration pattern of the DNA visualized, because it will change the length of the DNA fragments (RFLPs) detected by the radioactive probe (Figure 6–4).

DNA probes used to identify RFLPs can be derived from a large number of known chromosomal locations. Two types of strategies for linkage analysis have been employed. In one strategy, investigators use their complete set of chromosomal markers to systematically exclude increasingly larger regions of the genome as potential loci of a disease gene. By using a finer and finer DNA linkage map, investigators can close in on the disease gene and eventually identify it. This type of analysis has been used successfully to identify genetic linkages and, in some cases, the specific abnormal gene for an increasing number of human diseases, including cystic fibrosis.

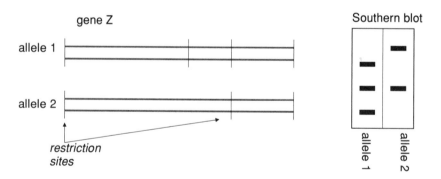

FIGURE 6–4. Schematic illustration of RFLP analysis. As a hypothetical example, assume two individuals have different alleles (alleles 1 and 2) for some gene *Z* and that the two alleles differ in DNA sequence such that a restriction enzyme recognition site located in allele 1 is lost from allele 2. In RFLP analysis, as shown in Figure 6–3, the total DNA from these individuals is digested with a restriction enzyme, the DNA fragments are separated by gel electrophoresis, and the fragments corresponding to gene *Z* are identified by Southern blotting using a radioactively labeled DNA probe containing the gene *Z* sequence. Because allele 2 has lost a restriction site, the Southern blots for the two alleles are different; that is, different-sized fragments of DNA are recognized by the gene *Z* probe. These different-sized fragments are referred to as restriction fragment length polymorphisms, or RFLPs.

An alternative strategy to identify disease genes is possible if good patho-physiological information is available concerning the disease. Such information provides clues as to the specific proteins that could potentially be abnormal under disease conditions. Genes encoding these proteins can be cloned and used as *candidate disease genes*. Polymorphisms identified within or near the site of these genes can then be used in a linkage analysis. The use of candidate genes can allow investigators to bypass the time-consuming systematic approach. The candidate gene approach has been used successfully in identifying the molecular abnormality underlying diabetes mellitus in certain families, namely, a mutation in the insulin receptor gene that renders the receptor protein relatively insensitive to insulin. Data also suggest that for a minority of pedigrees with familial Alzheimer's disease, the candidate gene strategy using the β-amyloid precursor protein may prove to be successful.

Linkage Analysis of Psychiatric Disorders

Despite some preliminary reports to the contrary, neither the systematic nor the candidate gene strategy of linkage analysis has been successful in psychiatry to date. One of the most dramatic initial findings was a report that a gene conferring vulnerability to bipolar disorder was linked to markers on the short arm of chromosome 11 in a large Old Order Amish pedigree. Segregation analysis had suggested that bipolar disorder was inherited in this pedigree as an autosomal dominant trait with incomplete (60%–70%) penetrance. This population is ideal for genetic study because of their large inbred families with a relative lack of confounding factors such as drug or alcohol abuse. (Inbreeding decreases the likelihood of heterogeneity.) The locus for bipolar disorder was reported to be linked to two polymorphic marker genes, the Harvey *ras* proto-oncogene and the insulin gene on the short arm of chromosome 11. The fact that these genetic loci are close to the gene for tyrosine hydroxylase led to considerable over-interpretation, for example, that bipolar disorder was related to abnormal cate-cholamine metabolism. However, further analysis of this same pedigree refuted the original claims. Two additional family members who did not possess the linked marker became affected (one with unipolar illness and one with late-onset bipolar disorder), and an additional branch of the original pedigree was studied that did not show evidence of linkage. At this time, it appears that either there is no linkage of bipolar disorder to the two markers on chromosome 11 or there is heterogeneity within the pedigree.

Linkage analysis of bipolar disorder is further complicated by reports of X linkage in certain Israeli pedigrees. X linkage can clearly be excluded in the Old Order Amish and several other pedigrees that have been studied. The possibility that bipolar disorder may be X linked in some families but not in others would suggest that abnormalities in different genes leading to different functional defects may give rise to a phenotypically similar behavioral syndrome. An important alternative hypothesis, strongly underscored by the recent experience with the Old Order Amish study, is that one or more of these linkage analyses is wrong, with evidence for linkage being due to misclassification of family members or to chance.

Similarly frustrating results have been obtained in linkage analysis of schizophrenia. Genetic linkage of schizophrenia to two genetic markers on the long arm of chromosome 5 was demonstrated in several British and Icelandic pedigrees. In contrast, no such linkage was found by analysis of multiple additional pedigrees.

In conclusion, the current difficulty in establishing linkage of psychiatric disorders to known genetic markers reflects, in part, our relative lack of knowledge of the disorders themselves and, in part, the likely complexity of the genetic factors involved. Nonetheless, molecular research strategies in psychiatry retain a great deal of promise. These strategies are among the topics of Chapter 7.

SELECTED REFERENCES

Baron M, Risc N, Hamburger R, et al: Genetic linkage between X-chromosome markers and bipolar affective illness. Nature (London) 326:289–292, 1987

Berrettini WH, Goldin LR, Gelernter J, et al: X-chromosome markers and manic-depressive illness. Arch Gen Psychiatry 47:366–373, 1990

Gusella J, Wexler N, Conneally P, et al: A polymorphic DNA marker genetically linked to Huntington's disease. Nature 306:234–238, 1983

Kelsoe JR, Ginns EI, Egeland JA, et al: Re-evaluation of the linkage relationship between chromosome 11p loci and the gene for bipolar affective disorder in the Old Order Amish. Nature (London) 342:238–243, 1989

Kennedy JL, Giuffra LA, Moises HW, et al: Evidence against linkage of schizophrenia to markers on chromosome 5 in a northern Swedish pedigree. Nature (London) 336:167–170, 1988

Merikangas KR, Spence A, Kupfer DJ: Linkage studies of bipolar disorder: methodologic and analytic issues. Arch Gen Psychiatry 46:1137–1141, 1989

Price RA, Kidd K, Weissman M: Early onset (under age 30 years) and panic disorder as markers for etiologic homogeneity in major depression. Arch Gen Psychiatry 44:434–440, 1987

Rice J, Reich T, Andreasen NC, et al: The familial transmission of bipolar illness. Arch Gen Psychiatry 44:441–447, 1987

Sherrington R, Brynjolfsson J, Petursson H, et al: Localization of a susceptibility locus for schizophrenia on chromosome 5. Nature (London) 336:164–167, 1988

Torgusen S: Genetic factors in anxiety disorders. Arch Gen Psychiatry 40:1085–1089, 1983

Wexler NS, Rose EA, Housman DE: Molecular approaches to hereditary diseases of the nervous system: Huntington's disease as a paradigm. Annu Rev Neurosci 14:503–530, 1991

Chapter 7

Toward a

New Psychiatric

Neuroscience

MOLECULAR BASIS OF
GENE-ENVIRONMENT INTERACTIONS

Both genetic and environmental factors play important roles in normal psychological development and in the pathogenesis of major psychiatric disorders. Family, twin, and adoption studies demonstrate that vulnerability to many major psychiatric disorders has a genetic component. Such studies also support the idea that genes contribute to many aspects of temperament, personality, and attitudes in addition to conferring vulnerability to disease. However, unlike some genetic disorders (e.g., Tay Sachs disease or Huntington's disease), the common major psychiatric disorders, as well as normal personality traits, do not result simply from the deterministic unfolding of genetic information. Studies of identical twins discordant for major psychiatric disorders demonstrate clearly that additional factors must interact with the genome to produce these illnesses.

Based on information presented in preceding chapters, we can begin to formulate possible mechanisms, at the molecular level, by which genetic and environmental factors combine to produce a mental disorder. It is also possible to begin to construct strategies by which these specific mechanisms can be studied. A working model of the molecular basis of gene-environment interaction is illustrated in Figure 7–1. Each person is endowed at conception with a unique

---

Text defined by vertical rules in the left margin involves advanced concepts and can be skipped by readers interested in a more general overview of the field, without loss of the overall message of the book.

genetic makeup, or genotype. Much of the remarkable diversity that exists among individuals is due to their distinct genotypes. This diversity reflects the large number of different alleles found within the human population at many, possibly most, genetic loci. At each meiosis, these alleles may recombine and segregate in novel ways to result in a unique combination of genes and hence a unique genotype.

Each cell in the body of a given individual contains the same genome with the same primary DNA sequences. However, only a fraction of all genes are expressed in any given cell type. It is this selective expression of genes and proteins in a cell that determines virtually every aspect of that cell's function. The different organs and different cell types within each organ originate during development by differential expression of this common genome. As a simple example, a particular neuron and a skin cell within any given individual contain the same complement of genomic DNA, but many of the genes that are being actively transcribed (expressed) in the neuron are not expressed in the skin cell, and vice versa. (The major exception to the rule of preservation of the primary DNA sequence occurs in T and B lymphocytes, in which the DNA sequences

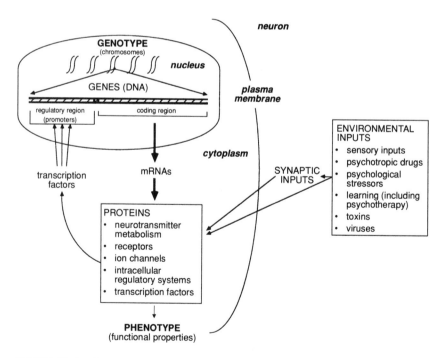

FIGURE 7–1.   Schematic illustration of gene-environment interactions. See text for discussion.

encoding T cell receptors and immunoglobulins are rearranged in a controlled fashion to produce the diversity needed to recognize a large number of antigens.)

Each individual's genotype interacts with the environment during development and, in fact, throughout life to produce that individual's unique phenotype. These interactions are achieved by a cell's (and organism's) environment influencing decisions as to which genes an individual cell will express at a particular time, as well as the level of that expression. The influence of environment on gene expression (plus some random variation) explains how individuals with identical genotypes (i.e., identical twins) still exhibit many phenotypic differences.

During development, many endogenous substances are known to exert a strong influence on gene expression in multiple target tissues. Prominent examples include steroid and thyroid hormones, growth hormones, trophic factors, and retinoic acid. Any external factor that alters these many endogenous regulators could potentially alter the development of the organism. Teratogenic drugs and chemicals, viruses, and nutritional deficiencies are all examples of exogenous environmental influences that may alter the normal patterns of gene expression during development and thereby produce marked effects on the phenotype of the individual.

Even after the overall phenotype (i.e., differentiation) of a cell has been stably determined during development (for some cells within the mammalian nervous system this point may not be reached until well after birth), environmentally induced changes in cellular structure and function continue to occur on a regular basis in virtually every cell type. These processes permit an adult organism to adapt successfully to a changing environment. Such adaptations have been long recognized for non-nervous tissues, and the most important molecular mechanisms involved have been shown over the years to be altered patterns of protein phosphorylation and/or of gene expression. Some environmental factors can lead to relatively isolated changes in the expression of particular genes: for example, ingestion of ethanol increases the expression of certain metabolic enzymes in liver cells. In other cases, complex effects on cell structure may occur that depend on changes in the expression of a relatively large number of genes: for example, those seen during hypertrophy of skeletal or heart muscle cells with exercise. In yet other cases, environmental stimuli may trigger cell division and actually alter the total number of cells: for example, exposure to an antigen may lead to clonal expansion of lymphocytes that recognize that antigen.

It has taken longer to recognize analogous long-term adaptive changes in the brain. Within the adult mammalian nervous system, neurons are postmitotic, that is, they no longer undergo cell division; however, they appear to exhibit every other type of adaptive change that has been recognized in peripheral tissues. In fact, such changes may be more marked and widespread in the brain, and more heavily influenced by diverse types of environmental factors, compared with most other organs. Incoming sensory information, psychotropic drugs, psychological experience and stressors, and psychotherapeutic interventions all produce long-term effects on the brain. The mechanisms by which psychotropic drugs influence brain function are becoming increasingly well established (as covered in Chapters 4 and 5); the most prominent mechanisms involve alterations in signal transduction pathways and neuronal gene expression in specific types of neurons in the brain. By analogy, it is almost certain that the long-term effects of all other types of environmental stimuli—even the most abstract environmental inputs such as spoken words—are mediated similarly; they likely activate specific neural circuits and the neurons within them. Synaptic events, in turn, influence intracellular second messenger and protein phosphorylation pathways, transcription factors, DNA regulatory elements, and, ultimately, the activation or repression of specific genes. The sum of such effects within large neural networks would then produce long-term changes in the overall functioning of the brain, and hence in the behavior of the individual as a whole (see Figure 7–1).

Individuals differ markedly in the way that they respond to specific environmental factors. For example, people show widely differing immune responses to various antigens, differences that reside both in their genotype (e.g., differences in human leukocyte antigen [HLA] type and other immune response genes) and in their history of environmental exposures (e.g., prior exposures to different antigens). Similarly, individuals vary greatly in response to new information, stressful events, psychotropic medications, psychotherapeutic interventions, and the like. Such differences are also likely to result from differences both in genes and in prior experience.

It will be a long time before we possess a detailed understanding of gene-environment interactions as they affect the brain, but, as discussed above, we have an understanding in principle of some of the major mechanisms involved. An understanding of the particular neural networks involved in each type of long-term change and identification of the specific genes and proteins within the critical neurons that are the targets of particular environmental stimuli are among the major challenges to modern psychiatric neuroscience. Ultimately, our ability to understand and manipulate the regulation of gene expression in the brain is a fundamental goal of a molecular approach to psychiatry.

How Environmental Factors Can Influence
Gene Expression in the Brain

Based on the concept that the environment regulates the long-term functioning of the brain by regulating intracellular signal transduction and neural gene expression, we will illustrate hypothetical mechanisms by which various types of environmental inputs might interact with specific genetic abnormalities to produce a mental disorder.

Physical environmental factors.   Several types of physical environmental factors have been hypothesized to be external triggers for the development of mental disorders, most notably schizophrenia, in genetically susceptible individuals. Hypothesized factors have included viruses, toxins, and physical damage to the nervous system (e.g., by anoxia or other injuries) in utero or during birth. Although there is not enough evidence to date to establish a role for such an etiologic factor in schizophrenia or any other disorder, it is possible to speculate as to how such factors might interact with specific genes to produce a mental illness.

Many types of viruses are known to infect neurons; these are often referred to as *neurotropic viruses*. Examples of neurotropic viruses include Epstein-Barr virus, herpes simplex virus, mumps virus, and the human immunodeficiency viruses. An individual's genetic makeup has a profound influence on the ability of a virus to infect a target cell, as well as the ways in which cell function changes as a result of the infection. In the hypothetical case of a mental disorder, appearance of the disorder would depend on 1) exposure to the virus, 2) genetic vulnerability to viral infection, and 3) genetically determined effects of the virus on the functioning of the infected neurons. With respect to the latter point, viral infection might be expected to alter the neuron's response to its various synaptic inputs or to lead to neuronal death. In either case, this could result in the mental disorder in question.

Toxins might be expected to work in analogous ways. An increasing number of toxic substances have been identified that alter the function of or kill specific neuronal populations in the brain. For example, certain heavy metals, plant toxins, and drugs (e.g., MPTP [1-methyl-4-phenyl-1,2,3,6-tetrahydropyridine], a contaminant in a "designer" drug of abuse) kill nigrostriatal dopamine neurons and thereby lead to parkinsonism. The ability of environmental toxins to contribute to development of a mental disorder would, as with viruses, depend on exposure to the toxin, on the genetically determined vulnerability of the neurons to the toxin, and on the subsequent death of the neurons or the adaptive responses of surviving neurons. It has been shown in animal models with lesions in the nigrostriatal pathway, for example, that the genes for multiple neuropeptides (e.g., the opioid peptide precursor proenkephalin) and the gene for the D_2 receptor become chronically activated in the striatum in response to the lesions.

Similarly, physical traumas sustained in utero or during birth might selectively influence or destroy certain neuronal populations in the brain. For example, neurons are known to vary greatly in their susceptibility to anoxia. The adaptive response of the brain to an injury probably varies among different individuals, and this variation may be partly genetically determined.

Two additional complexities must be taken into consideration to develop the strongest possible heuristic model of the role of physical damage in producing a mental illness via interactions with the genome. First, until this point we have considered cases in which a single environmental factor would contribute to a mental disorder. In reality, multiple factors might combine in complex ways with multiple genetic loci to lead, ultimately, to the expression of a particular illness. Second, it is important to emphasize that an environmental injury sustained early in life might lead to the development of a mental illness years, perhaps decades, later as the nervous system matures.

This scenario has been suggested by a number of investigators, including Goldman-Rakic, Weinberger, and Benes. Such a delay between initial injury and clinical symptoms can be explained by the fact that certain classes of neurons may only become functionally important at later stages in development—for example, at adolescence—such that loss, injury, or alterations in the activity of those neurons early in life become clinically apparent only at some later point. Adolescence is an active time in brain development in part because of the appearance of high levels of sex steroids, which appear to produce marked effects on behavior through altered expression of multiple neural target genes. This is particularly intriguing given the peak onset of a number of neuropsychiatric disorders (e.g., schizophrenia) during adolescence and young adulthood. It has been speculated, for example, that a perinatal injury to the brain or childhood infection might selectively destroy certain neurons within the prefrontal cortex, which would lead to floridly abnormal cortical function (e.g., schizophrenic symptoms) only when those neurons are recruited to full functional activity during adolescence. In thinking about the etiology of schizophrenia, such a scenario, which includes a critical role for the environment, is particularly attractive given the observation that when a member of a monozygotic twin pair has schizophrenia, the co-twin is concordant for schizophrenia only 40%–50% of the time.

Psychological experience and trauma.   From the time of Freud, it has been widely presumed that psychological experiences influence not only normal personality development, but also the appearance of at least some mental disorders later in life. This view is still widely accepted, and it would be hard to imagine that this would not be the case. However, it has been difficult to demonstrate in a convincing fashion that particular patterns of life experience or particular psychological traumas lead specifically to particular mental disorders. Unilaterally environmentalist views of the etiology of psychiatric disorders, still held by many psychiatrists, are unlikely to prove correct. Although many psychodynamic theorists acknowledge a role for "inborn temperament" in the development of character and of mental disorders, this concept is often left in the background. Instead, the pathogenesis of psychiatric disorders is commonly understood entirely in terms of the causal role of certain psychological experiences at particular developmental stages. In other words, the all-too-prevalent norm in the clinical practice of psychiatry is for causal explanations of mental symptoms to be based narrowly on a chain of environmental and developmental circumstances. When they are testable, explanations of this sort generally fall short. A rather gross example is that they fail to explain the marked similarities in personality traits that typify identical twins raised apart and the marked differences in outcomes among children faced with similar developmental circumstances. Genetic determinist models are equally deficient in explanatory power, failing to address, for example, identical twin pairs who are discordant for personality traits or for the presence of major mental illnesses.

How might psychological experience interact with a person's genome to influence character traits or the development of a mental disorder? Life experience is perceived by an individual through sensory neurons—for example, sights by the retina and spoken words by the auditory system. This information is first analyzed in primary sensory areas of the cerebral cortex, then in unimodal sensory association cortices, polymodal association cortices, and limbic brain areas, with a wave of successive brain regions recruited to analyze, interpret, synthesize, and act on the original sensory inputs. Depending on both internal and external circumstances, such as the individual's state of arousal, these processes will be modulated by ascending monoamine neurons and other modulatory systems. Such perception, interpretation, response, and modulation are mediated via synaptic connections among a large number of individual neurons. As discussed in Chapters 2 and 4, such synaptic activity leads not only to immediate neuronal outputs, but under certain circumstances also initiates cascades of long-term adaptations in synaptic activity (mediated via changes in protein phosphorylation and gene expression) that would produce prolonged, and some relatively stable, alterations in brain function, including memories. Such changes in brain function, then, might alter the individual's response to subsequent environmental events.

Early in life, experiences might be expected to exert important and perhaps permanent influences on brain function if particular experiences occur (or fail to occur) at times when relevant systems are undergoing development. For example, it has been shown in animal models that critical periods in the development of primary visual and somatosensory cortices occur in early postnatal life.

During such periods, synapses that are actively used are stabilized and inactive synapses are selected against. After the end of those critical periods, the resulting patterns of synaptic connections are relatively resistant to further change, barring catastrophic damage to the nervous system. Although at present there is no direct evidence for critical periods of heightened plasticity in brain regions that might be correlated with the development of personality traits (e.g., association cortices or the limbic system), the possible existence of such periods might explain the apparent importance of early experience in establishing relatively stable personality traits, patterns of self-understanding, or patterns of response to other people or stressful situations.

We have been considering the role of the environment as if it were an independent factor, but it should be recalled that an individual's genotype would be expected to exert a profound influence on his or her response to particular experiences and behavioral cues in combination, of course, with prior experience. There are an extremely large number of genes, many still undiscovered, whose protein products set the intrinsic excitability of specific neurons or the relative strengths of their many synaptic connections. Such genes would thereby alter the responsiveness of specific neurons to various environmental inputs. Thus, genotype might determine, in part, which experiences are salient to a particular individual (e.g., stressful, exciting, rewarding, aversive) and which are ignored. Clearly, genes and environment interact in a complexly intertwined fashion in which genes partly create and select the environment experienced by the developing individual and in which the environment affects the expression of genes.

Pharmacotherapies and psychotherapies.   There are a large number of therapeutic measures available to psychiatrists to treat mental illness. These treatments are often divided into two major categories: somatic (pharmacological and electroconvulsive therapies) and psychosocial (the different individual, group, and family therapies, which may be insight oriented, cognitive, or behavioral). Both classes of interventions can be effective in treating particular mental disorders, depending on the individual and the nature of the disorder. The best treatment for a particular disorder remains a matter of empirical research. Our understanding of psychiatric disorders is too primitive to rely on any theory, no matter how compelling, to determine which treatments should be effective for a given disorder. Where both pharmacotherapies and psychotherapies have proved to be effective, the clinician has maximum choice in matching a treatment to the needs of the individual patient. For example, it appears that in the treatment of *mild* depression, antidepressant medications and certain cognitive therapies specifically designed for the treatment of depression may be equally efficacious. How can such widely differing therapeutic approaches result in similar outcomes, in this case successful treatment of depression? Our view is that both measures produce their therapeutic effects in ways that will ultimately prove to be similar. Despite acting through markedly different neural pathways initially, any therapies that effectively treat the core symptoms of depression will eventually have to produce similar long-term changes in the same sets of neurons. Of course, the overall experience of psychotherapy or of taking a medication will, in addition to these basic effects (i.e., treating the depression), potentially leave other very different impressions on the nervous system and the psyche, but even these differential effects result from the production of long-term changes in the functioning of neurons and neural circuitry. Whether a particular medication or a particular psychotherapeutic intervention can help for a given psychiatric disorder must depend on whether the treatment in question effectively produces the appropriate changes within the appropriate neural pathways.

Considerable attention was given in Chapter 5 to the mechanisms by which psychotropic drugs regulate neural plasticity. Although much remains to be learned, it is probable that psychotropic drugs such as antidepressants, antipsychotic drugs, and lithium attenuate the symptoms of mental illness by a cascade of events in which acute alterations in neurotransmitter-receptor systems and intracellular messenger pathways produce slower-onset, long-lasting adaptive changes in target neurons through the regulation of protein phosphorylation and gene expression. These adaptations may result in long-term changes in synaptic function both at the level of the synapse itself (e.g., via altered levels of neurotransmitter synthetic enzymes, neuropeptides, or neurotransmitter receptors) or at the level of the efficacy of the neurotransmitter receptor–mediated signal on the postsynaptic cell (e.g., via altered levels of postreceptor signal transduction proteins). By analogy, it is likely that psychosocial interventions also attenuate the symptoms of mental illness by acutely influencing the activity of specific neural and intracellular pathways in the brain and, consequently, by producing longer-lasting changes in the function of specific neurons via the regulation of protein phosphorylation and neuronal gene expression.

An important goal is to identify the types of neural changes that lead to therapeutic improvement and then to use the primary intervention (drug or psychosocial) that produces those changes in the safest, most rapid, and most effective way. Identification of such therapeutic changes would also provide novel ways to screen for more effective treatments, as will be discussed later in this chapter.

Nature versus nurture.   When posed as a rigid dichotomy, the "nature versus nurture" question leads to false conclusions and confusion. However, the question is valid and important when reconstrued as an attempt to understand the means by which gene-environment interactions produce various traits and illnesses. The contributions of genetic and environmental factors to normal personality development and to the development of mental illness probably vary considerably among diverse traits and illnesses. It should eventually be possible to improve understanding of the nature of these contributions with advances in twin, adoption, and human genetic studies and molecular genetic analyses. In principle, it should be possible to identify individual genes that affect normal psychological traits or confer vulnerability to mental illness, as well as at least some of the specific environmental factors that influence their expression. Indeed, the analysis of environmental factors is likely to prove analogous to the analysis of genes, in that we may be able to identify a few of the major contributors to particular phenotypes, but may not be able to identify a large number of minor contributors. In practice, however, for traits or disease vulnerabilities that depend on more than a few genes and environmental factors, this type of analysis may not be possible in the short run.

Achieving an understanding of gene-environment interactions in more than superficial terms will be exceedingly difficult. This is illustrated by the probability, already alluded to earlier, that genes affect the relevant environment for psychological development as much as the environment affects the expression of genes. Assume, for example, that an infant's temperament is determined largely by genes (subject, of course, to the uterine environment). The early developmental environment provided by the child's parents results not only from the parents' characters, means, wishes, and plans a priori; the way parents interact with a child is also conditioned by the effect of the child on the parents. A smiling, interactive child is likely to elicit different responses from most parents than an irritable or disinterested child. In this way, a child's genotype as expressed by his or her temperament conditions the environment, which then feeds back on the child's genotype during development. This sort of complexity makes the modeling of gene-environment interactions in human behavior particularly challenging.

When construed in such a sophisticated way, investigation of the nature versus nurture question should lead to important advances in psychiatry. However, this dichotomy must be distinguished from another often posed in the field of psychiatry, a dichotomy that is often framed as "biological versus psychological." This latter dichotomy assumes a Cartesian separation between body and mind; it is ultimately confused and misleading. This view discounts the possibility of effective causal interactions between psychological and environmental factors on the one hand and between the brain and genome on the other. The impact of experience on brain function is relegated to a black box and, after a bit of lip service, is generally ignored. In fact, it should be clear from this discussion that all psychological inputs are ultimately recorded in the brain and that all psychological outputs reflect biological processes. The more critical point is that there are specific biological mechanisms that we, as psychiatrists and neuroscientists, are beginning to understand that can provide the missing causal links. There is, of course, a valid (and unanswered) philosophical question of the precise relationship of consciousness to brain function. However, it is not necessary to await better solutions to that age-old question to see that the Cartesian position assumed by many psychiatrists is untenable, unhelpful, and at times just silly.

It is common in psychiatry, for example, to construe certain disorders (e.g., personality disorders) as environmental and developmental in origin, and as a result—so the Cartesian inference goes—to be treated with psychological therapies. In contrast, other disorders (e.g., manic-depressive illness) are generally construed as biological in origin and are therefore to be treated with somatic therapies. These formulations are nothing short of absurd. Both personality disorders and mood disorders represent the product of gene-environment interactions, and either psychological or somatic therapies could in principle be effective for both. Despite the absurdity of this type of Cartesian inference, it is reified by current psychiatric nosology in which personality disorders are placed on a separate "diagnostic axis" from other psychiatric disorders.

Remarkably, it is often assumed that if a symptom can be treated with a medication, it must be biological rather than psychological in origin. This may be the most absurd expression of the biological versus psychological dichotomy. In fact, anxiety or fright produced by language and ideas can be treated by benzodiazepines, just as the anxiety following a spontaneous panic attack may be mitigated by finding a safe place or person.

We want to underscore that we are not arguing for a reductionism that would diminish the importance or validity of psychological explanations. (When someone is asked why he hates his mother, an answer based on quantum mechanics or even neural circuitry is likely to be less explanatory than an answer at the psychological level.) What we mean is that there are causal bridges among the molecular, the neural, and the psychological levels of analysis, and that it is a central task of the basic science of psychiatry to elucidate these bridges. Only then can we develop a full understanding of mental disorders with a view to developing the most effective treatments.

The complexity of the brain and of human psychology make this a staggeringly difficult task. However, the experimental difficulty of achieving an understanding of the brain at this level should not detract from the importance and validity of this goal: urgently needed advances in the diagnosis, treatment, and prevention of severe mental disorders depend on the identification of specific neuronal and intracellular factors involved in the pathophysiology of specific diseases. We will now discuss some currently available experimental strategies that can be used to work toward this ambitious goal.

OVERVIEW OF PSYCHIATRIC
NEUROSCIENCE

As is clear from earlier chapters in this book, much remains to be learned about the pathophysiology of most psychiatric disorders and the important clinical actions of psychotropic drugs. Indeed, there is a growing sense in the field that improved knowledge can only be obtained through fundamentally new approaches in psychiatric neuroscience.

Most prior efforts to understand the brain from a psychiatric point of view have been hampered, with some important exceptions, by taking a very narrow view of brain function. Psychiatric neuroscience, and especially the field of neuropsychopharmacology, has too often focused exclusively on synaptic events (e.g., neurotransmitter metabolism—synthesis, storage, release, reuptake, and degradation—and receptor binding), without extending its vision upward to the level of neural networks or downward to the level of the molecular events occurring after binding of neurotransmitters or drugs to their receptors.

These studies in biological psychiatry have tended to take a very limited endocrine-like view of the brain instead of a neurobiological view. That is, the functions of particular neurotransmitters were not generally considered in the context of specific neural pathways or of multiple receptor subtypes, but neurotransmitters were considered to act more globally to produce related biological effects on target tissues (as is the case for a hormone). For example, depression was conceptualized as a norepinephrine or serotonin deficit or schizophrenia as a state of dopamine excess. In fact, the brain is not well described in terms of the isolated functioning of individual neurotransmitters. Neurotransmitter systems are complexly interacting so that changes in firing rates of neurons containing one neurotransmitter will alter the release and functioning of other neurotransmitters in multiple pathways. Moreover, the concept of a neurotransmitter deficit (e.g., "a serotonin deficit") is not straightforward: different serotonergic projections have a panoply of different functions at different receptor subtypes, and, as a result, the serotonin system exerts markedly different biological effects on its many target neurons. It is likely, then, that psychiatric disorders are not caused by generally abnormal levels of particular neurotransmitters or numbers of particular neurotransmitter receptors, but are caused by disorders in the regulatory properties of particular neuronal cell types that secondarily affect the actions of multiple neurotransmitter and receptor systems.

Even more striking in biological psychiatry has been the frequent failure to look beyond the receptor level for additional sites of drug action and disease pathophysiology. Altered synaptic function—for example, altered patterns of neurotransmitter release and receptor binding—produces many complex changes in target neurons in addition to rapid alterations in electrical activity. The fact that the important clinical actions of most psychotropic drugs require their chronic administration indicates that these longer-term adaptive changes in brain function, and not the acute changes in electrical activity per se, underlie crucial aspects of drug action.

To a certain extent, the myopia of biological psychiatry to date has reflected real experimental limitations in studying brain function. There has also been a clear failure, until very recently, to take full advantage of the powerful methods of molecular biology and modern neuroscience. Psychiatric neuroscience today should utilize advances in these rapidly developing fields to extend earlier investigations from a narrow focus on the synapse to analyses of neural systems on the one hand and studies of postreceptor signal transduction events occurring within neurons on the other.

Consideration of "systems neurobiology" is beyond the scope of this book. Readers are encouraged to pursue this subject through other sources. Certainly it is critical that the types of molecular analyses described below be complemented by parallel efforts to elucidate the function of neural networks within which molecular and cellular mechanisms operate.

STRATEGIES FOR A MOLECULAR APPROACH TO PSYCHIATRIC NEUROSCIENCE

The general strategy we favor for psychiatric neuroscience in the coming decades is to combine the search for psychiatric disease genes, as described in Chapter 6, with basic studies of the nervous system. The genetic and neurobiological approaches are complementary, and both are necessary to achieve the needed advances. Basic neuroscience can help identify realistic candidate genes for genetic studies and is necessary if the functions of disease genes, identified by any method, are to be analyzed. The full ramifications of discovering a gene conferring vulnerability to a psychiatric disorder can only be realized by determining the functional and regulatory properties of the protein products of the normal and abnormal alleles of that gene. Similarly, basic studies of the brain, in and of themselves, cannot easily identify the actual genes contributing to the etiology of psychiatric disorders and must therefore be complemented by genetic studies.

We view two aspects of basic neuroscience as particularly relevant in this endeavor. First is the use of psychotropic drugs as molecular probes of nervous system function. This reflects the view that studies of psychotropic drug action continue to provide the best information about the aspects of normal brain function most relevant to psychiatry and, ultimately, about brain processes involved in mental disorders. Moreover, there is ample evidence that drugs influence many of the same cellular and molecular substrates in laboratory animals as they do in humans; therefore, findings at the molecular level in laboratory animals can probably be extrapolated to humans.

Second are attempts to elucidate the mechanisms that underlie gene-environment interactions occurring during development and beyond. In one sense, psychotropic drugs can be seen as prototypical environmental factors producing changes in gene expression, because we would expect other types of environmental factors, including psychological experience, to influence brain function via similar types of mechanisms. It will be important to consider the whole gamut of environmental factors that may influence brain development and plasticity, and to consider whether there are critical periods of enhanced plasticity in brain regions relevant to the development of personality traits and psychiatric disorders.

Clearly, investigations of the role of experience and behavior in neural plasticity will not be straightforward, but here, too, significant progress is possible. Animal models are available for drug addiction that make it feasible to investigate the genetic and environmental factors that influence drug reinforcement and craving, which are critical determinants of drug addiction. For example, genetic strains of rats that exhibit different susceptibility to drug addiction provide useful models with which to investigate the types of genes that contribute to the differences in behavior between strains, as well as the environmental factors that influence the expression of these genes. Attempts could also be made to identify the genes and proteins whose expression is altered under particular paradigms of stress. One related question is whether antidepressant drugs and certain behavioral stressors used in animal models of depression regulate the same molecular pathways but in an opposite manner. Identification of such shared molecular actions could even be used to develop better animal models of depression and related disorders.

The identification of disease genes, in combination with the tools of molecular neurobiology, may finally permit us to understand, in detail, the pathophysiology of psychiatric disorders and should contribute to the development of more effective treatments for mental illness. Such studies may also lead to the first objective diagnostic criteria in the field of psychiatry. In addition, the availability of psychiatric disease genes will permit us to identify individuals at risk for psychiatric disorders. Prospective longitudinal studies of such individuals, in combination with findings from basic neuroscience, may help identify particular environmental factors that protect against mental disorders and other factors that increase the risk of mental disorders. Ultimately such research should contribute to prevention of the disorders in question.

The Search for Psychiatric Disease Genes

It is possible, in principle, using molecular genetic techniques, to discover genes that confer vulnerability to psychiatric disorders and even genes that contribute to normal psychological traits (see Chapter 6). Study of DNA polymorphisms in families with psychiatric disorders was initially greeted with great excitement by psychiatric researchers, based on success in identifying tightly linked markers (e.g., in Huntington's disease) or actual disease genes (e.g., in cystic fibrosis) for nonpsychiatric disorders. Early reports claimed to identify restriction fragment length polymorphisms (RFLPs) that cosegregated with vulnerability to bipolar disorder and to schizophrenia in certain pedigrees. However, initial enthusiasm has given way to increased skepticism, as these early reports have gone unconfirmed and some have even been disconfirmed.

As described in Chapter 6, analysis of DNA polymorphisms is a powerful approach with great promise, but it is critically dependent on our ability to classify patients as either "affected" or "unaffected" by the disorder in question. Such definitive diagnoses are currently not possible for the major psychiatric disorders. Psychiatric genetics is also complicated by the observation that many disorders do not show clear Mendelian patterns of inheritance. This may be due to reduced penetrance and variable expressivity of genes, but also perhaps to the involvement of multiple interacting genes. An additional complication is the likelihood that phenotypically indistinguishable psychiatric disorders may be genetically heterogeneous in etiology or due to environmental causes.

One way to improve diagnostic measures would be to identify pathophysiological markers of psychiatric disorders. Such markers could then be used to identify more homogeneous subgroups of patients, who could be studied along with their families by DNA polymorphism analyses, with a greater potential for success. Here too, psychiatry faces an exceedingly difficult problem. Pathophysiological studies of psychiatric disorders, such as those using pharmacological and neuroendocrine challenges or neuroimaging, have yielded only small and often nonreproducible differences between affected and unaffected individuals. This difficulty may be due in part to the fact that populations picked out by phenotypic diagnostic criteria, such as criteria in DSM-III-R, may be pathophysiologically heterogeneous. A circular problem should now be obvious: the availability of genetic markers would permit pathophysiological studies to focus on etiologically homogeneous patients, but without pathophysiological subgrouping of the sort that theoretically could be provided by challenge studies and neuroimaging, it may be very difficult to identify homogeneous patients for genetic studies in the first place.

Clearly, a great deal of work remains to be done in the selection of patients for both types of studies and in delineating the diagnostic boundaries of particular disorders. Promising advances are offered by the field of neuroimaging. Most neuroimaging studies of psychiatric disorders to date have, by necessity, focused on static morphometric measurements or rather low-resolution measurements of blood flow or oxygen utilization. Blood flow and oxygen utilization are correlated with neuronal activity and could therefore, in principle, be related to abnormal information processing or abnormal neuronal outputs in the brain. Abnormalities of neuronal activation have been posited in schizophrenia, panic disorder, and other psychiatric disorders based on current technologies, but the low resolution of these technologies has made it impossible to draw specific pathophysiological inferences from them at present. However, improvements in magnetic resonance imaging (MRI) methods and the development of new radiolabeled pharmacological probes are likely to make it possible to study specific proteins in the brains of living, awake people.

Two of the major imaging methodologies are single photon emission computed tomography (SPECT) and positron-emission tomography (PET). The major difference between SPECT and PET is the different types of radioisotopes that are used. Another difference is the better resolution currently possible for PET, although improved SPECT cameras may decrease this difference. In both techniques, a radioactively labeled compound is administered to a person systemically, and the radioactivity is then detected and quantitated over time in computerized cross-sections of the brain. This makes it possible to study the level, affinity, and anatomical localization of the proteins in the brain to which the radiolabeled compound binds. SPECT and PET can be combined with MRI to enable even more exact anatomical localization of the visualized proteins. By use of these imaging techniques, it has been possible to image D_2 receptors and $GABA_A$ receptors in specific regions of the human brain. It is anticipated that in the future it will become possible to image a large number of neurotransmitter receptors and specific subtypes of receptors, as well as neurotransmitter reuptake proteins and intracellular signal transduction proteins (e.g., G proteins, protein kinases, glucocorticoid receptors).

An additional technology of great promise is magnetic resonance spectroscopy (MRS), which can detect the levels of particular ions and of some proteins with a reasonable degree of quantitative precision. It may eventually be possible to determine levels of particular proteins in the brains of patients and their family members to define pathophysiological markers of mental disorders.

Finally, ultrafast MRI scanning is being developed that will allow real-time depiction of blood volume (and, therefore, presumably brain activity) with far higher spatial and temporal resolution than blood-flow studies with PET. In combination, these various neuroimaging technologies may markedly improve psychiatric diagnostics and thereby facilitate psychiatric genetics studies.

It may also be possible to develop improved physiological and pharmacological challenge studies. Pathophysiological studies of patients should be combined with similar analyses of their affected and unaffected relatives as well as with analyses of unrelated control populations. It is possible that such methods will enable the identification of some clinically unaffected individuals who exhibit the same pathophysiological abnormalities as their affected relatives. In this vein, abnormal extraocular movements among psychotic patients and their family members have been proposed as a physiological marker of genetic vulnerability to schizophrenia, but a convincing connection between abnormal eye movements and the pathophysiology of schizophrenia remains to be demonstrated. Nonetheless, success with this strategy could dramatically improve the accuracy of psychiatric genetics studies.

Identification of Candidate Genes

The genetic approach described to this point in this chapter assumes that we have no prior knowledge of the proteins (or genes) responsible for the pathophysiology of mental disorders and must therefore search for linkage of disorders to "anonymous" DNA probes. For reasons described earlier, the systematic use of anonymous probes in psychiatry has met with considerable difficulty. Instead of systematically excluding linkage of a disease to anonymous probes scattered throughout the genome, linkage to specific candidate genes could be tested. A *candidate gene* is defined as a gene believed a priori to be involved in the pathophysiology of the disorder. Not only is this approach more efficient than the systematic approach in that it requires only a very limited linkage analysis, it is also statistically more powerful. This is because, by definition, a successful candidate gene will be tightly linked to the disease locus. Tight linkage should compensate for the diagnostic problems described (i.e., it will tolerate some statistical "noise").

However, the candidate gene approach only makes sense when there is a good pathophysiological theory that implicates a specific gene. The candidate gene approach has not been used successfully to date in psychiatry because, lacking adequate pathophysiological theories, it has not been possible to identify true candidate genes. The possibility of using candidate genes to establish genetic linkage (and therefore the etiology of the disorder) underscores the need for improved pathophysiological understanding of psychiatric disorders in molecular terms.

An optimistic view of the interaction of molecular studies of pathophysiology with genetics is supported by recent successes in identifying disease genes in other, albeit simpler, illnesses—certain forms of diabetes mellitus, for example.

Diabetes, like psychiatric illnesses, is a clinical syndrome with different genetic abnormalities involved in different families. A major breakthrough was the identification of a phenotypic subtype of diabetes in certain families in which the illness involved resistance to insulin action in target tissues. Another important breakthrough resulted from basic biochemical and molecular biological studies over the past decade that elucidated many of the precise molecular pathways by which insulin produces its effects in target tissues. It was found that in addition to a binding site for insulin, the insulin receptor possesses protein tyrosine kinase activity required for insulin action. Based on this knowledge, it was demonstrated that, in some families, diabetes is caused by mutations in the insulin receptor that abolish its protein tyrosine kinase activity. It has also been found that some of the actions of insulin on its target tissues are mediated through a specific insulin-sensitive glucose transporter protein. In laboratory animals, certain forms of experimental diabetes can be caused by alterations in the transporter protein that render the protein less responsive to regulation by insulin, raising the possibility that similar alterations may be involved in some other cases of human diabetes. As knowledge of the pathways underlying insulin action becomes more complete, it is likely that the affected genes in an increasing number of families with diabetes will be identified.

Analogous studies in psychiatry can lead to the identification of genes that contribute to specific psychiatric disturbances. A given psychiatric syndrome may be associated with a large, but finite, number of different genetic abnormalities among different pedigrees. Related clinical and laboratory studies could lead to the identification of specific types of environmental factors that interact with particular disease genes to produce a given mental disorder and of the precise molecular mechanisms involved. Together, these types of advances should have a profound effect on the future course of psychiatry.

Experimental Approaches to Identification of Proteins and Genes Involved in Psychotropic Drug Action and Mental Disorders

Several powerful methods are now available to identify specific genes, proteins, and regulatory processes involved in the action of psychotropic drugs and potentially involved in mental disorders. Such methods may eventually yield promising candidate genes that can be studied for linkage to psychiatric disorders and used as tools for the development of novel drugs.

Initial identification of proteins with potential roles in psychiatric disorders could involve demonstrating their 1) regulation by specific psychotropic drugs or other relevant environmental perturbations, 2) anatomical specificity—that is, expression or drug regulation in specific brain regions implicated in a given psychiatric disorder, and/or 3) differential expression or regulation in genetically inbred strains of laboratory animals that serve as models for psychiatric disorders.

Many of the experimental methods used to identify and characterize such proteins have been mentioned throughout this book; we will now describe these strategies and potential applications in general terms. Clearly, these represent only a sampling of the many powerful methods currently available in psychiatric neuroscience.

Studies of neural signaling proteins. Signal transduction proteins are known to be the targets of the acute and chronic actions of many psychotropic drugs on specific neuronal populations in the brain (see Chapter 5). For example, specific neurotransmitter synthetic or degradative enzymes, reuptake transporters, and receptors, as well as G proteins, second messenger enzymes, and other components of intracellular messenger pathways, appear to play important roles in the adaptive responses of neurons to chronic drug action and by analogy to other types of environmental factors. Constituents of signal transduction pathways also represent potential sites of pathophysiological abnormalities in patients with psychiatric disorders. For these reasons, as more is learned about them, genes encoding certain neural signaling proteins may prove to be reasonable candidate genes for studies in psychiatric genetics.

One interesting development in recent years from molecular cloning studies (see Figures 7–2 and 7–3) is the existence of a staggering number of signaling proteins in the nervous system. In these studies, investigators have searched for closely related but nonidentical proteins by hybridizing fragments of DNA (Figure 7–2) that encode a particular protein (e.g., a G protein–linked receptor) to a library of DNA fragments (Figure 7–3) under so-called low-stringency conditions. These are conditions that tolerate a degree of mismatch between complementary sequences. (*Mismatch* refers to lining up of the nucleotides A or T across from C or G in double-stranded DNA instead of A across from T and C across from G, as described in Chapter 1).

If these studies are successful, a variety of related clones will be identified. By such methods it has been found that the brain contains, for example, *at a minimum*: 15 G protein α subunits, 15 GABA$_A$ receptor subunits, hundreds of G protein–linked receptors, and multiple subtypes of particular protein kinases, ion channels, etc. (See Chapter 2.) Scores of G protein–linked receptor-like molecules that have been molecularly cloned have yet to have their ligands defined. One such unknown was recently identified as the cannabinoid receptor (cannabinoids are the active substances in marijuana); its endogenous ligand remains unknown. Recall that of the approximately 100,000 genes found within the human genome, at least 30,000 are expressed solely or primarily in the brain. Additional cloning studies are needed to identify still more subtypes of signaling proteins in the nervous system, and basic molecular neurobiological studies are needed to characterize these numerous proteins with respect to their biochemical, anatomical, physiological, and pharmacological properties, as well as their potential role in the pathophysiology of mental disorders.

Identification of novel drug-regulated proteins by protein phosphorylation. Because only a small fraction of the proteins expressed within neurons have been identified and characterized to date, it is also critical to utilize more open-ended approaches to discover novel targets of drug action. Such novel proteins can be revealed by protein phosphorylation studies, which take advantage of the paramount role played by protein phosphorylation in the regulation of neuronal function (see Chapters 2 and 4). In such experiments, brain extracts (e.g., from control and from drug-treated animals) are phos-

FIGURE 7–2 *(at right).* **Schematic illustration of molecular cloning methods.** To study genes or produce DNA probes for hybridization experiments (such as those described in Figure 6–3), large amounts of the genes or other DNA fragments of interest must be produced. This is accomplished by molecular cloning. Molecular cloning requires restriction endonucleases that can specifically cut DNA (see Figure 6–2), enzymes that can join DNA fragments (DNA ligase), and a *cloning vector.* Cloning vectors are either bacterial *plasmid* DNA or *bacteriophage* virus DNA that can replicate autonomously in bacteria such as *Escherichia coli* (*E. coli*). Autonomous replication means that the plasmids and bacteriophages can replicate (reproduce) without integrating into the single large circular chromosome of *E. coli*. Plasmids are small DNA circles that carry only a few genes, whereas bacteriophages are much larger. Plasmids used in cloning were originally engineered from antibiotic-resistance plasmids found naturally in bacteria; these plasmids encode enzymes that break down antibiotics. Plasmids and bacteriophages that are useful for cloning yield many copies of the vector per bacterial cell.

As shown in the figure, a DNA fragment of interest is prepared using restriction enzymes. The cloning vector—a plasmid is shown—is cut with the same restriction enzymes so that the fragment of interest (called the *insert*) and the vector will have complementary ends that can anneal together to reconstitute a region of double-stranded DNA. The mixture of the DNA fragment to be cloned and the cut vector is treated with DNA ligase, which joins the annealed ends. The ligated plasmid is then introduced into *E. coli,* where it replicates. Most commonly used cloning vectors contain an antibiotic-resistance gene (e.g., for ampicillin resistance); by growing *E. coli* in medium containing ampicillin, investigators can thereby select for only those bacteria that have taken up the plasmid. The *E. coli* containing recombinant plasmids are then grown, after which time the plasmids are separated based on their different densities from the *E. coli* chromosomal DNA and *E. coli* proteins by centrifugation. An investigator can obtain milligram quantities of a single DNA fragment from a standard plasmid preparation using 1 liter of *E. coli* suspension.

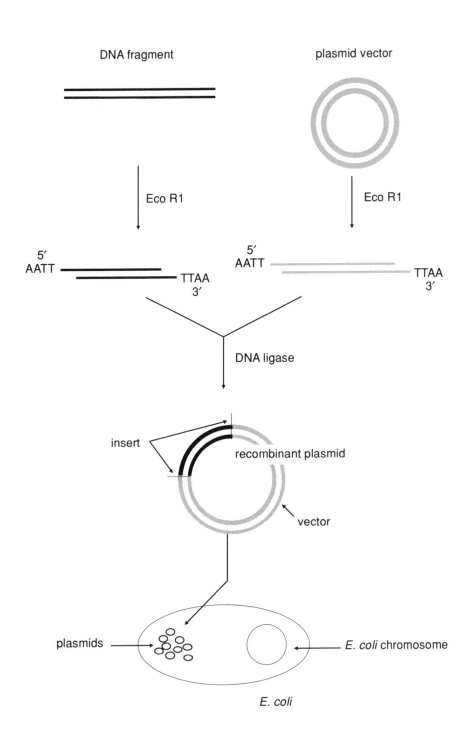

phorylated by protein kinases and radioactively labeled ATP. The protein kinases transfer a radioactive phosphate group from the ATP to their specific substrate proteins. Individual radioactively labeled phosphoproteins are then resolved by one-dimensional SDS-polyacrylamide gel electrophoresis, which separates proteins on the basis of their size (i.e., molecular weight), or by two-dimensional gel electrophoresis, which separates proteins on the basis of both their charge and size. Individual phosphorylated proteins are identified by autoradiography, that is, by exposing resulting gels to X-ray film. Examples of drug-regulated phosphoproteins demonstrated by one- and two-dimensional electrophoresis are shown in Figure 7–4. Such initial identification of novel drug-regulated phosphoproteins is then followed by their extensive characterization. This approach has been used with great success by a number of laboratories to identify proteins that play important roles in the regulation of neuronal function, in psychotropic drug action, and most recently in the pathophysiology of Alzheimer's disease.

Identification of novel drug-regulated proteins by subtraction cloning.
Novel drug-regulated proteins can also be revealed by subtraction cloning, which enables the identification of messenger RNAs (mRNAs) not present or

FIGURE 7–3 *(at right).*   **Schematic illustration of complementary DNA (cDNA) library construction.** Figure 7–2 illustrates the cloning of a single DNA fragment. A *library* of clones can also be prepared; such a library contains a mixture of inserts representing all of the genes expressed in a given tissue or cell type.
    To construct a cDNA library, a particular tissue (e.g., a brain region) is dissected, homogenized, and chemically extracted to yield pure RNA, which can be further purified to yield only messenger RNA (mRNA). A sample of the mRNA of a tissue represents all of the genes that are being transcribed (i.e., expressed) in that tissue. For example, a sample of hippocampus would contain mRNA encoding GABA_A receptor subunits, but not mRNA encoding hemoglobin. Total mRNA can be treated with a viral enzyme—reverse transcriptase (so named because it "reverse transcribes" RNA into DNA)—in the presence of nucleotide building blocks to yield cDNA copies of each RNA.
    Synthetic DNA sequences can then be added to the end of each of the linear cDNAs to provide "sticky ends" that will anneal with a restriction enzyme–cut vector. After ligation into the vector (as shown in Figure 7–2), the recombinant plasmids (or bacteriophages) are used to transform *Escherichia coli* (*E. coli*). Conditions are such that each *E. coli* contains only one plasmid or bacteriophage and therefore only one cDNA insert. The *E. coli* are spread on an agar plate containing ampicillin (to suppress any growth of bacteria that have not taken up the plasmid or bacteriophage). Each bacterium grows into a colony, each of which contains multiple copies of a single gene expressed within the starting tissue. A library is "screened" for particular genes using probes that will detect particular sequences by complementary base pairing. In the figure, a plasmid is shown for simplicity, although bacteriophage vectors are also commonly used for library construction.

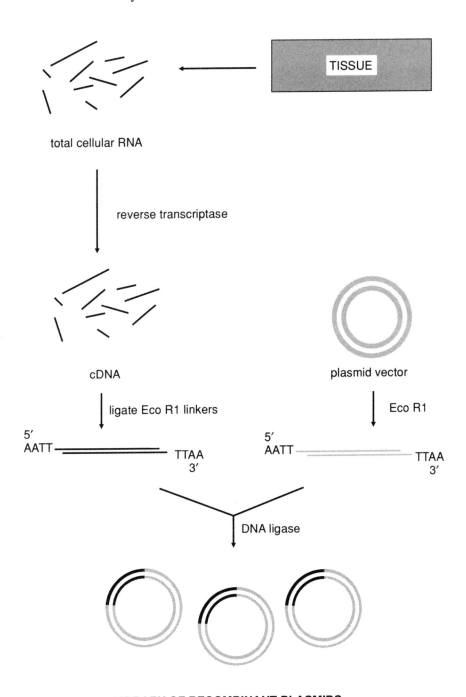

LIBRARY OF RECOMBINANT PLASMIDS

present at much lower levels in one tissue sample compared with another tissue sample. In this technique, mRNA is isolated from two sources of tissue, for example, from a specific brain region of untreated rats and from rats treated chronically with a psychotropic drug. The goal is to identify mRNAs whose expression is drug regulated. In the example depicted in Figure 7–5, complementary DNA (cDNA) is synthesized from the mRNA derived from drug-treated animals. This cDNA is then mixed with a large excess of mRNA from control animals. By the principle of complementary base pairing, the cDNAs that have a complement within the mRNAs will hybridize to them, whereas cDNAs that do not hybridize to mRNA remain single stranded and potentially represent drug-induced species. These cDNAs are then isolated and cloned. An analogous subtraction using cDNA from control animals and mRNA from drug-treated animals yields potential drug-repressed species.

Subtraction hybridization thereby involves the identification of drug-regulated proteins, with no prior knowledge of their functional or structural properties. A clue to the function of such "subtracted" cDNAs can be derived from determining their DNA sequence, which would indicate whether they have been cloned previously in other studies or whether they might belong to a family of receptors, G proteins, protein kinases, etc. Basic molecular neurobiological studies are then required to further characterize the proteins and to establish their role in the mechanism of action of the original drug treatment. There are many methods of subtraction cloning, all of them challenging and requiring great care. Despite the technical difficulty, however, this method has great potential to identify previously unknown drug-regulated genes.

Studies of the regulation of gene expression.   It is important to emphasize that a protein identified (in studies of neural signaling proteins, protein phosphorylation, or subtraction cloning) as drug regulated may not represent the etiological site of psychiatric pathophysiology; such proteins may be removed from the biochemical "lesion" by one or more steps. Even if the

FIGURE 7–4 *(at right)*.   **Examples of one- and two-dimensional electrophoretic analysis of proteins.** The figure illustrates the use of protein phosphorylation to study candidate genes in psychiatry. Specifically, it shows the identification of morphine-regulated phosphoproteins in *A)* the rat locus coeruleus by one-dimensional SDS-polyacrylamide gel electrophoresis, and *B)* the ventral tegmental area by two-dimensional gel electrophoresis. These specific studies are discussed in more detail in Chapter 5. IEF = isoelectric focusing.

   Source.   Panel B is from Beitner-Johnson D, Guitart X, Nestler EJ: "Neurofilaments and Mesolimbic Dopamine System, I: Common Regulation by Chronic Morphine and Chronic Cocaine in the Rat Ventral Tegmental Area." *Journal of Neuroscience* 12:2165–2176, 1992. Used with permission.

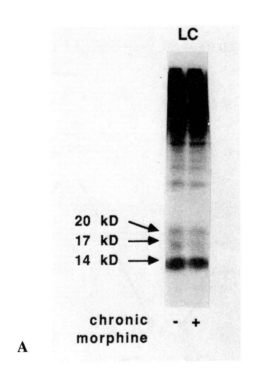

A

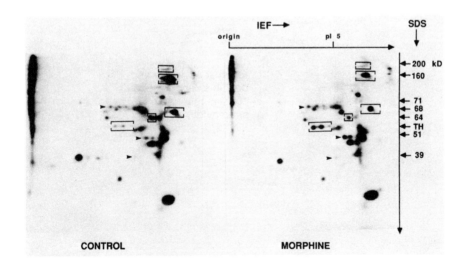

B

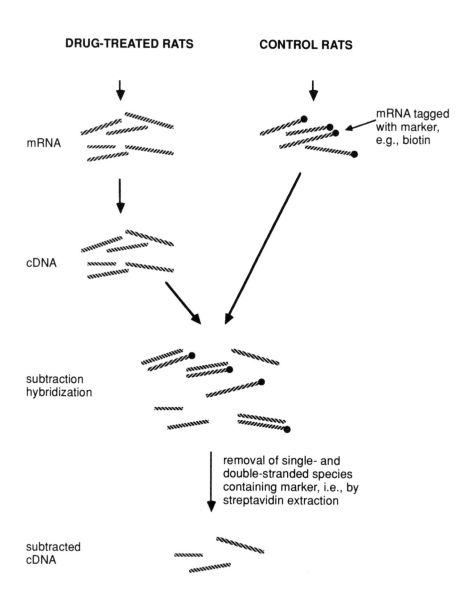

FIGURE 7–5. Schematic illustration of subtraction hybridization. See text for discussion. mRNA = messenger RNA. cDNA = complementary DNA.

protein is itself involved in the etiology of a mental disorder, the predisposition to the disorder may not reside in an abnormality of the protein itself, but in processes that regulate its function or genetic expression. Indeed, it would appear to be more likely that a genetic abnormality contributing to the development of a mental disorder lies in such a regulatory process rather than in the actual sequence of a major protein itself. This view is based on the observation that most psychiatric disorders begin at some discrete time, such as during adolescence or adulthood. If a major structural or signaling protein (e.g., a neurotransmitter receptor or ion channel) were itself abnormal, patients might be expected to manifest a disease phenotype from birth. In addition, many syndromes, such as mood and anxiety disorders, are episodic, with periods of illness spontaneously remitting with the passage of time, or proving more rapidly reversible with appropriate treatment. This reversibility also favors abnormalities in regulatory processes—for example, an abnormality in the regulation of the expression of a receptor or ion channel, as opposed to an abnormality in the primary sequence of that protein, per se. This possibility underscores the importance of studying the intracellular messenger systems, transcription factors, and DNA promoter elements (see Figure 4–2) that control the genetic expression and function of proteins and genes identified in the studies involving neural signaling, protein phosphorylation, and subtraction cloning.

Studies with transfection and transgenic models.   Many of the proteins identified by low-stringency screening of cDNA libraries, by cloning of regulated phosphoproteins, and by subtraction hybridization will yield genes and proteins of unknown identity and function. Such genes might also be identified by linkage analysis using anonymous probes. The amino acid sequences of the proteins, which can be deduced from their DNA sequences, may suggest a function for the genes, but more definitive determination of their function requires that they be returned to eukaryotic cells under controlled circumstances. This can be accomplished by one of two major methods, transfection and production of transgenic animals.

In transfection studies, genes are introduced into eukaryotic cells in tissue culture (Figure 7–6). Gene expression requires an active promoter (see Chapter 4) and generally the entire region of DNA that codes for the protein itself. To study the function of an unknown gene product, its cDNA (which largely represents the gene's coding region) can be fused to a highly active promoter, for example, a promoter derived from a virus. This fusion gene can be introduced or "transfected" into some eukaryotic host cell, where it will be transcribed and its protein product subsequently produced. If, for example, based on sequence homology, the gene is thought to encode an unknown G protein–linked receptor, it can be transfected into tissue culture cells that will then transcribe the gene, produce the protein, and express it on their surface membranes. The transfected cells can then be used in radioreceptor binding assays to try to identify the ligand of the unknown receptor. Such methods have been used to establish the function of many cloned receptors, and analogous methods have been used to study the function of many other types of cloned genes.

Transfection can also be used to study the regulation of gene expression rather than the protein product of the gene in question. This involves analysis of the function of the promoter and other regulatory regions within the gene. This form of analysis is based on alteration (mutation) of regulatory elements in vitro followed by transfection. What is then observed is the ability of the altered regulatory regions to drive transcription. Because it is the regulatory region of the gene that is under study rather than its protein product, the coding

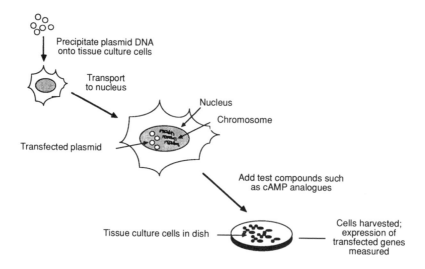

FIGURE 7–6. Schematic illustration of transfection methods. Transfection involves the introduction of DNA into eukaryotic cells. DNA of interest is transfected either as a linear fragment or ligated into a plasmid. (DNA can also be introduced ligated into a virus, in which case the term *infection* may be used instead of *transfection*.) The figure shows the transfection of plasmid DNA. In one commonly used method, plasmid DNA is precipitated out of solution with calcium phosphate, and the precipitate is layered on eukaryotic tissue culture cells that adhere to the bottom of a dish. The cells take up the DNA and, by a process that is not understood, transport it to the nucleus where transcription factors bind to it, allowing it to be expressed. The results of expressing the DNA of interest can then be assessed.

region of the gene is generally replaced with a "reporter" gene, which codes for the synthesis of an easily assayed protein product. Reporter genes in common use are bacterial chloramphenicol acetyltransferase (CAT) or β-galactosidase or firefly luciferase. Assay of the reporter gene product then reflects the level of gene expression being directed by the regulatory sequences under study. An example of this type of analysis is shown in Figure 7–7.

Transfection studies are limited by the types of cells that can be grown in culture and by the fact that, for neural systems, the connectivity of the brain is lost. To study the function of a gene in the context of the whole brain, the most important current method is the production of transgenic mice. This method involves harvesting mouse embryos at the one-cell stage before the male and female pronuclei are fused. The gene of interest is injected into one of the pronuclei, and the embryo is implanted in the oviduct of a foster mother mouse. This *transgene* is integrated into the mouse's genome a certain percentage of the time, with the result being a mouse expressing the gene of interest. Because the transgene is contained within all cells of the mouse, including its germ line, it can be passed on to future generations. An additional form of transgenic technology allows the "knock out" of endogenous genes. For unknown genes identified as described in previous sections of this chapter, the construction of transgenic animals may be the most promising way of finding out the normal function of the gene as well as its contribution to disease pathophysiology.

This would appear to be the case for psychiatric disease genes identified by linkage analysis with anonymous probes. It would also appear to be the case for proteins first identified, by protein phosphorylation and subtraction cloning (as described earlier in this chapter), as drug regulated. For this latter case, transgenic mice can be engineered to express altered levels of a certain protein shown to be involved in the mechanism of action of a particular drug, for example, a drug of abuse. The behavioral properties of the transgenic animals (e.g., their drug preference or craving) can then be studied. It should be pointed out that these types of experiments represent the forefront of experimental procedures in molecular neurobiology and have been carried out only very recently. Some of these experiments may even remind one of science fiction. However, recent technical advances have now made such studies feasible for wide application to psychiatry.

THE FUTURE OF PSYCHIATRY

Until very recently, the basic science of psychiatry has lagged behind that of most other medical specialties in identifying etiological factors and pathophysiological mechanisms of disease processes so as to improve diagnosis and

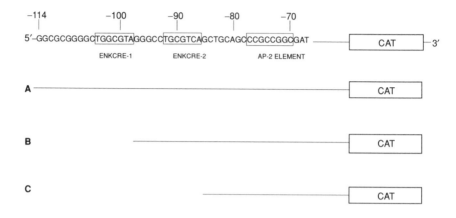

FIGURE 7–7.   Deletion analysis of a DNA regulatory region; the proenkephalin gene is used as an example. The *top row* shows the known DNA regulatory elements *(boxed sequences)* that constitute the proenkephalin enhancer (see Chapter 4 for definitions of promoter terminology). The relevant DNA sequences are shown; the rest of the 5′ flanking region of the gene is shown as a *solid line*. The coding sequence of the gene has been replaced by a reporter gene, chloramphenicol acetyltransferase (CAT). The numbers above the DNA sequence refer to the number of bases upstream of the transcription start site. Alterations can be made in the 5′ flanking region of this construction, and CAT expression can be assayed after transfection into eukaryotic cells. *Rows A–C* illustrate a deletion analysis, which is the initial approach used to analyze a promoter.

Row *A* represents a construction containing the entire enhancer sequence of the proenkephalin gene. When it is transfected and the cells are treated with cyclic AMP, the gene is fully activated as measured by increased expression of CAT activity.

In *Row B*, one of the DNA regulatory elements (ENKCRE-1) has been deleted, and when this construction is analyzed, the response of the gene to cyclic AMP is diminished 10-fold.

The deletion shown in *Row C* removes a second regulatory element (ENKCRE-2) in addition to the first. The gene is now inactive despite a remaining element (AP-2), which is apparently not strong enough to work on its own. The gene can now be further analyzed by mutating individual bases within the response elements. Even such small mutations can alter the ability of transcription factors to bind to their respective DNA elements. This type of analysis was used to define the boundaries of the regulatory elements in the proenkephalin gene promoter that mediate the gene's responsiveness to cyclic AMP. These response elements, termed *ENKCRE-1* and *ENKCRE-2,* bind the AP-1 (Fos and Jun) families of transcription factors (see Chapter 4). The AP-2 element, which presumably mediates the responsiveness of the proenkephalin gene to other cellular signals, is so named because it binds the "activator protein-2," or AP-2.

treatment. These advances in general medicine, most achieved in the latter half of this century, have followed largely from basic biomedical investigations of the cellular, subcellular, and molecular mechanisms underlying the genetic and environmental factors responsible for the cause, manifestation, course, and treatment of a large number of medical illnesses.

The basic concept of the medical model in psychiatry is that mental disorders are diseases of the brain and, therefore, are entirely analogous to diseases of other organ systems. Identification of specific genetic abnormalities that contribute to mental disorders and delineation of the mechanisms by which environmental factors influence the expression of those genes should revolutionize diagnostic, treatment, and preventive aspects of psychiatric practice.

Molecular advances in psychiatry should lead to an improved understanding of the pathophysiological basis of particular disease states and, ultimately, to the development of safer, more efficacious treatments. Objective diagnostic tests should permit the accurate establishment of specific psychiatric disorders, with implications for the choice of treatment and communication of meaningful prognostic information to patients and their families. Eventually, such advances may even make it feasible to prevent specific mental disorders.

In this book, we have attempted to illustrate how an improved understanding of the brain's neurotransmitter-receptor systems, intracellular signal transduction pathways, and genetic regulatory mechanisms might lead to such a promising future for psychiatry.

SELECTED REFERENCES

American Psychiatric Association: Diagnostic and Statistical Manual of Mental Disorders, 3rd Edition, Revised. Washington, DC, American Psychiatric Association, 1987

Andreasen NC: Brain imaging: applications in psychiatry. Science 239:1381–1388, 1988

Bouchard TJ, Lykken DT, McGue M, et al: Sources of human psychological differences: the Minnesota study of twins reared apart. Science 250:223–250, 1990

Caskey CT: Disease diagnosis by recombinant DNA methods. Science 236:1223–1229, 1987

Friedmann T: Progress toward human gene therapy. Science 244:1275–1281, 1989

Garvey WT, Huecksteadt TP, Birnbaum MJ: Pretranslational suppression of an insulin-responsive glucose transporter in rats with diabetes mellitus. Science 245:60–63, 1989

Goldman PS: Functional development of the prefrontal cortex in early life and the problem of neuronal plasticity. Exp Neurol 32:366–387, 1971

Goldman PS, Mendelson MJ: Salutary effects of early experience on deficits caused by lesions of frontal association cortex in developing rhesus monkeys. Exp Neurol 57:588–602, 1977

Gusella JF: Location cloning strategy for characterizing genetic defects in Huntington's disease and Alzheimer's disease. FASEB J 3:2036–2041, 1989

Hanahan D: Transgenic mice as probes into complex systems. Science 246:1265–1275, 1989

Nestler EJ, Greengard P: Protein Phosphorylation in the Nervous System. New York, Wiley, 1984

Odawara M, Kadowaki T, Yamamoto R, et al: Human diabetes associated with a mutation in the tyrosine kinase domain of the insulin receptor. Science 245:66–68, 1989

Travis GH, Sutcliffe G: Phenol emulsion-enhanced DNA-driven subtractive cDNA cloning: isolation of low-abundance monkey cortex-specific mRNAs. Proc Natl Acad Sci U S A 85:1696–1700, 1988

Weinberger DR: Implications of normal brain development for the pathogenesis of schizophrenia. Arch Gen Psychiatry 44:660–669, 1987

Index

*Page numbers in **boldface** type refer to tables or figures.*